NEUROMUSCULAR MECHANISMS FOR THERAPEUTIC AND CONDITIONING EXERCISE

Edited by

Howard G. Knuttgen, Ph.D.
Boston University

University Park Press
Baltimore · London · Tokyo

UNIVERSITY PARK PRESS
International Publishers in Science, Medicine, and Education
233 E. Redwood Street
Baltimore, Maryland 21202

Copyright© 1976 by University Park Press
Second printing, February 1980

Typeset by The Composing Room of Michigan Inc.
Manufactured in the United States of America by Universal Lithographers,
Inc., and The Maple Press Co.

Library of Congress Cataloging in Publication Data
Main entry under title:

Neuromuscular mechanisms for therapeutic and conditioning
exercise.

Bibliography: p.
Includes index.
1. Exercise—Physiological effect. 2. Muscles.
3. Exercise tests. 4. Exercise therapy. I. Knuttgen,
Howard G.
QP301.N46   612'.76   76-25248
ISBN 0-8391-0954-7

Contents

Contributors

Robert B. Armstrong, Ph.D.
Assistant Professor of Health Sciences and Biology
Sargent College of Allied Health Professions and
College of Liberal Arts, Boston University
Boston, Massachusetts 02215

L. Howard Hartley, M.D.
Associate Professor of Medicine
Harvard University Medical School
Boston, Massachusetts 02115

C. David Ianuzzo, Ph.D.
Associate Professor of Physical Education and Biology
Departments of Physical Education and Biology,
York University, Ontario, Canada

Howard G. Knuttgen, Ph.D.
Professor of Physiology
Sargent College of Allied Health Professions and
Graduate School of Arts and Sciences, Boston University
Boston, Massachusetts 02215

Whitney R. Powers, Ph.D.
Professor of Anatomy
Sargent College of Allied Health Professions and
School of Medicine, Boston University
Boston, Massachusetts 02215

Roger G. Soule, Ph.D.
Associate Professor of Health Sciences
Sargent College of Allied Health Professions, Boston University
Boston, Massachusetts 02215

Preface

This book was written for the purpose of providing, in a single volume, up-to-date information on the structure, nervous control, and function of skeletal muscle and of establishing the foundation for the application of muscular exercise as a precision tool in testing, conditioning, and rehabilitation. The authors have assumed a basic understanding of human anatomy and physiology on the part of the reader. Further, the reader should have an appreciation for the present limitations of the science of exercise physiology, and must accept the fact that many basic and practical questions remain to be answered. The information provided in this text should help the readers to answer many questions, but, at the same time, it will raise many new questions for consideration.

The volume begins with a discussion of how muscle cells are innervated and controlled. Then, an intensive review of muscle ultrastructure is presented, followed by a complete coverage of the energy release mechanisms available to, and utilized by, the muscle cell. The following two chapters cover, in general, the physiological responses of the total human organism to various types of physical exercise, the manner in which exercise must be utilized, and programs designed to fulfill specific objectives. The final section covers the very specific application of exercise as a testing and conditioning modality for the heart patient.

The authors hope that the information selected for inclusion and the manner in which the information is presented will constitute both an aid to learning and an invitation to the reader to add to the body of knowledge about exercise and the human organism.

Definition of Terms

A variety of systems of terminology are found in the literature related to physical exercise, a situation that can lead to confusion on the part of a reader. To promote effectiveness of communication, the authors have held to the definitions and interpretations of key terms as presented below:

Muscle Contraction: The attempt of muscle stimulated by efferent impulses to develop tension and shorten the longitudinal axis. Whether the muscle does shorten, is maintained at a set length, or is forcibly stretched during contraction is dependent upon the external resistance.

Exercise: Any and all physical activity involving movement, maintenance of posture, or expression of force by muscles. Exercise is synonymous with physical effort, physical activity, and exertion. In activity involving skeletal movement, the muscle may perform a shortening (concentric) contraction or be overcome by the resistance and perform a lengthening (eccentric) contraction. When muscle activity results in no skeletal movement, the contraction is termed isometric.

Exercise Intensity: A specific level of physical activity being maintained that can be defined in terms of work per unit time (power level), sustained isometric force, or repeated isometric contractions at a particular level of force.

Work: Force expressed through a distance but with no limitation on time.

Power: Force expressed through a distance per unit of time. In our discussion, the force may be generated by the human muscle and/or an external source.

Strength: The maximal effective force that can be voluntarily exerted in a specific movement (a specific condition for which type of contraction, velocity, and angle of joint are described).

Endurance: The time limit of a person's ability to maintain either a specific isometric force or a specific level of power.

Fatigue: The inability of a physiological process to continue functioning or of a person to maintain a predetermined intensity of exercise.

Skeletal muscle activity results in forces being exerted on the body's skeleton. As a result, postures are maintained in spite of the pull of gravity, movements are brought about, or force is exerted on external objects. All forms of such muscular activity can be included in the single term *exercise.*

When muscle cells are stimulated, they display the capacity to generate tension or force. *Force* is what tends to change the state of rest or motion in matter. When force is expressed through a distance, *work* is performed. In an isometric contraction, force is exerted, but, as there is no movement, no distance is involved and no physical work is performed. Also, the concept of work has no limitation of time. The force can be expressed through the distance slowly or rapidly, and the work performed remains the same.

Power is the time rate at which work is performed. To calculate power production, one must know the time interval involved, the average force generated, and the total distance through which the force was expressed.

Skeletal muscle fibers, when stimulated via nervous impulses, attempt to shorten themselves longitudinally. In this way, they generate tension or force between their skeletal attachments. If the force generated is greater than that of the resistance, the muscle shortens (*concentric* contraction) and work can be performed on external objects or on the body itself. When the force is insufficient to produce movement, the contraction is termed *isometric* and no work is produced. If an external force overcomes the effective force of the active muscle, work is performed on the muscle as it is stretched (*eccentric* contraction).

The total time to fatigue that muscles can maintain continuous activity involving the three types of contraction is termed *endurance.* In isometric contractions, no work is performed and the exercise can be defined in terms of force (tension) and time. In concentric contractions, endurance can be defined in terms of the length of time a certain level of external power production can be maintained (e.g., as measured in Watts or kg/m/min). In eccentric exercise, endurance would be the time to fatigue at a certain power level, in which work is being done on the muscle.

Strength is the term employed for the maximal effective force (actually *torque*) that can be generated in a voluntary movement. The conditions under which "strength" of a movement is determined must be precisely defined, because strength varies according to such factors as:

1. The type of contraction—concentric, isometric, or eccentric.
2. The joint angle at which it is determined.
3. The velocity of movement in phasic contraction (concentric or eccentric).

Neuromuscular Mechanisms for Therapeutic and Conditioning Exercise

Nervous System Control of Muscular Activity

Whitney R. Powers

EVOLUTION OF CONDUCTION IN THE NERVOUS SYSTEM

To fully understand and comprehend the mechanisms responsible for the activation and control of skeletal muscle, one must consider the evolutionary functional adaptations that have given rise to a more efficient nervous system capable of interpreting and responding to multiple types of sensations. Man, with great ability to reason, has evolved through three major changes: centralization; segmentation; and encephalization, the most sophisticated neural configuration of any living creature.

Even in encephalization there is a relationship between the size of a specific animal's cerebrum and its importance in the evolutionary adaptation of the animal's life cycle. One has only to compare a series of vertebrate brains to visualize the gradual "cephalic shift" (encephalization) of functions from the lower brain stem to the cortex of man (Figure 1). As man's cortex (neopallium) was developed, other less important neural structures became smaller. Yet, once a neural structure becomes part of the vertebrate nervous system it remains in higher forms, but in a reduced size and not necessarily with a reduced functional significance.

The highest development in man, the cerebral cortex, has been assumed to control the more caudally located sensory and motor projection systems of the thalamus, basal ganglia, brain stem, and cerebellum. The elaborate development of the neocortex by the sensory projection system has made it necessary to establish a new efferent (motor) projection

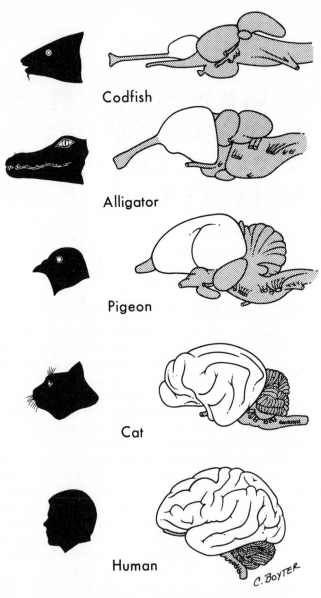

Codfish

Alligator

Pigeon

Cat

Human

ENCEPHALIZATION

Figure 1. A representative series of vertebrate brains showing the cephalic shift (encephalization) from the brain stem to the cortex of man.

system of the highest order to interconnect the lower neural mechanisms. These new sensorimotor neural connections established a means by which the pre-existing neural mechanisms of the brain stem could establish, through integration, control, and feedback, a smooth voluntary muscle movement both for groups and individual muscles. Thus we have established a mechanism in which the gross movements and fine prehension movements of activities of daily living have established the highest level of integration.

It has been held for the past several decades that the highest level, the cerebral cortex, through its efferent projection (pyramidal system) was responsible for the initiation and control of fine voluntary movements, and other extrapyramidal systems (basal ganglia, brain stem, cerebellum) were responsible for gross patterns of movements. In 1958, Herbert Jasper and his colleagues (26) established the method of single nerve fiber recordings from the motor cortex of monkeys. From this technique, Kemp and Powell (27) and Evarts (14, 16) have reported that single fiber recordings coupled with EMG (electromyography) recordings showed that, prior to motor activity in skeletal muscle, nerve action potentials could be recorded from the cortex, cerebellum, basal ganglia, and thalamus. It was therefore concluded that the cerebellum, basal ganglia, thalamus, and cerebral cortex interact in controlling skilled movements, in contrast to the previous assumption of a hierarchial level of control by the cortex.

These more recent studies verified Hughlings Jackson's original view, as presented in 1897, of the relationships of different divisions of the nervous system to one another and to the various parts of the body. It is essential, therefore, that we abandon our older concept of cerebral cortex motor control and return to Jackson's concept of total integration.

The advantage of the more complex neocortex of higher mammals is the perfection of neural mechanisms for the discrimination and storage of previous sensory and motor experiences. The *Homo sapiens* of future generations will continue to show evolutionary developments because of advances in environment, nutrients, and training, but it is appropriate at this time to examine the current understanding of our nervous system as a controlling mechanism.

GENERAL CONTROL OF BODY FUNCTIONS

The functional control of the various anatomical structures by the central nervous system can be analyzed through three major divisions:

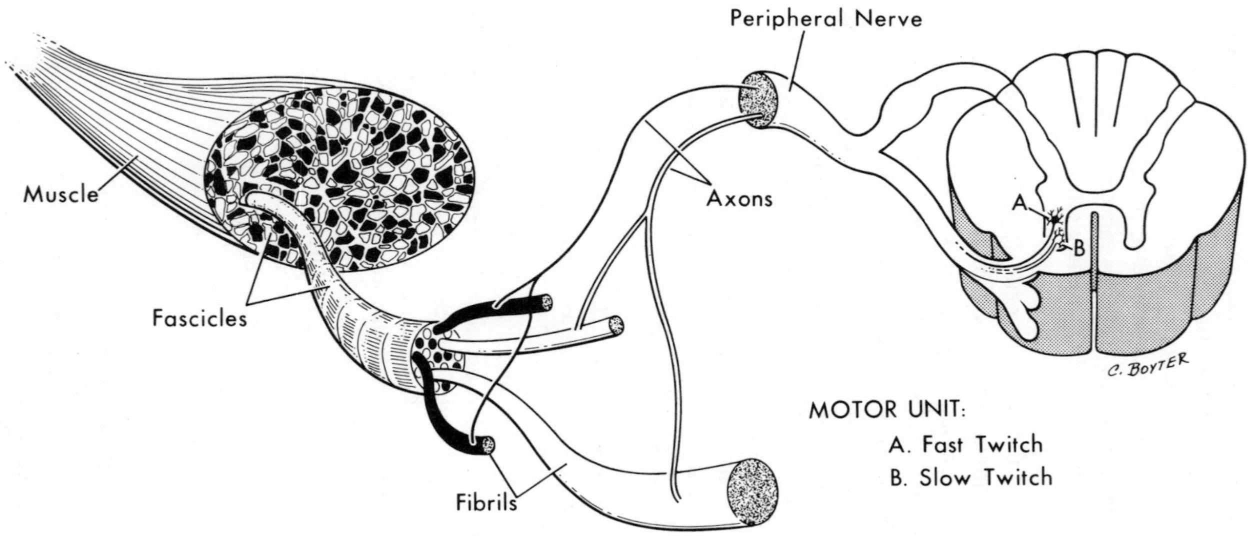

Figure 2. Schematic drawing of the components of a motor unit: the anterior horn cell, its axon, and all the muscle fibers the cell innervates.

Division 1. Vital Functions

Vital functions, e.g., respiration, cardiac activity, vasomotor control, and secretion, are preprogrammed and autonomically controlled by internal body requirements.

Division 2. Reflex Functions

Reflex functions are receptor-effector reactions to the environment, some of which are protective. Examples are: withdrawal responses, upright posture, cephogyric responses, coughing reflex, sneezing reflex, vomiting reflex, etc.

Division 3. Voluntary Functions

Our voluntary control of activities of daily living, which is achieved by the integration of suprasegmental (brain and brain stem) and segmental (spinal cord) connections, is described according to recent findings mentioned earlier.

We are addressing our attention to Division 3 functions, namely voluntary control of skeletal muscle. In order to gain a better insight into the controlling mechanism of skeletal muscle, we must begin by dividing this complex component into its basic parts.

MOTOR UNIT

Because the motor unit depends on an output-input configuration (15), it is logical to begin with the effector component, the motor unit. A motor unit is defined as consisting of an anterior horn cell, its axon, and all the muscle fibers innervated by it (Figure 2). Basmajian (6) and Grant and Basmajian (9) refer to these units as "little motors." Indeed they are, because they produce activity that, given the proper feedback system, can be made purposeful. The more power that is needed, the more motor units that are recruited into activity.

It must be pointed out that, without the abundance of sensory units that each segment of the spinal cord is endowed with, the motor units (little motors) would be ineffective and uncoordinated. The sensory unit consists of a dorsal root ganglion cell, its axon, and the particular receptor ending, i.e., extrinsic or intrinsic, it has developed according to its anatomical location in the body (Figure 3).

It is interesting to note that the entire sensory and motor unit components of the body carry an estimated 2½ million fibers to and from the central nervous system (CNS) with unequal distribution from

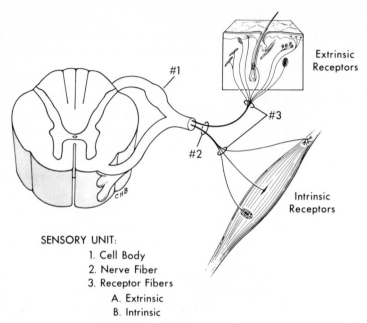

Figure 3. Schematic drawing of the components of a sensory unit: dorsal root ganglion cell body, its axon, and the two receptor dendrite locations (intrinsic and extrinsic).

side to side. Of this total, approximately 2 million are recognized as sensory fibers and the remaining ½ million as motor fibers.

In any single segment, the ratio of sensory to motor varies from 2:1 to 10:1 depending on the innervation ratio of that particular segment. In 1931, Clark (10) defined the innervation ratio as the ratio of motor nerve fibers supplying a muscle to the total number of muscle fibers in the muscle. Motor units with the lowest innervation ratios and the smallest diameter muscle fibers are found in muscles responsible for fine-precision movements. Motor units with the high innervation ratios and large diameter muscle fibers are found in muscles responsible for power and gross movements.

In a more detailed analysis of the effector mechanisms of the body and hence the motor units, there are two major types of motor units recognized: alpha motor units and gamma motor units. It is probable that we can further subdivide the alpha motor units, which are responsible for the innervation of skeletal muscle (so-called extrafusal fibers), into two subdivisions: alpha fast-twitch neurons and alpha slow-twitch neurons.

The fast-twitch neurons are characterized by large neurons, large axons (heavily myelinated), and innervation of a large number of pale ("phasic") muscle fibers. These pale motor-unit fibers are responsible for movements producing power and mass activity.

The slow-twitch neurons are characterized by small neurons, small axons (lightly myelinated), and innervation of a small number of red ("tonic") muscle fibers. These red motor-unit fibers are responsible for substantiated contractions, such as those supporting the body in the upright position.

Gamma motor units, in contrast to the alpha motor neurons, innervate the intrafusal muscle fibers, which are found inside the muscle spindles (a part of the intrinsic feedback mechanism of skeletal muscle). Approximately 30% of the fibers in the ventral root of the spinal cord are small somatic efferent fibers destined for the intrafusal muscle fibers of the muscle spindle. These fibers are smaller, and therefore conduct more slowly than the axons to the extrafusal muscle fibers.

The fusimotor or gamma efferent fibers can be subdivided into two groups (gamma 1 and gamma 2) on the basis of: stimulation threshold, conduction velocity, nerve cross-sectional size, and structure of terminal endings.

Boyd (8) claimed that the gamma 1 (γ_1) fibers innervate the nuclear-bag fibers with plate endings and the gamma 2 (γ_2) fibers innervate the nuclear-chain fibers with diffuse endings (Figure 4). Barker and co-workers (3, 4) agree that there are two types of efferent endings but believe that gamma motor fibers are not restrictive to one intrafusal fiber type. Kennedy (28) reported that certain motor axons have been found to branch and innervate both the intrafusal and extrafusal muscle fibers. These fibers have been termed beta fibers; yet all spindles do not exhibit a beta fibers type of motor innervation. At this time, beta fiber functional significance is unknown and the intrafusal fiber innervation is still controversial. Although the functional organization of the muscle spindle still remains to be solved, it is second in complexity only to the eye and ear, since it serves as a constant monitor to the length of muscles as well as to the speed of stretching, both of which are necessary for the proper CNS control of muscular contractions.

It is interesting, however, to speculate concerning the possibility of a relationship between the functional subdivisions of the gamma efferents and the subdivisions of the alpha motor neuronal pool innervation. The phasic and tonic alpha motoneurons would correspond to fast twitch and slow twitch extrafusal fiber motor units (as differentiated by time to peak

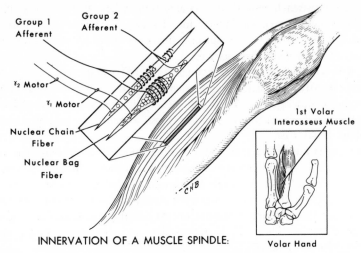

INNERVATION OF A MUSCLE SPINDLE: Volar Hand

Figure 4. Simplified concept of the innervation of a mammalian muscle spindle.

tension of the component fibers). A comparison of the dynamic and static components of the muscle spindle and the gamma system to the alpha cell innervation to extrafusal fibers can be summarized as follows:

Dynamic	Static
Gamma 1 motoneuron	Gamma 2 motoneuron
Gamma 1 fusimotor fiber	Gamma 2 fusimotor fiber
Nuclear bag intrafusal fiber	Nuclear chain intrafusal fiber
Primary sensory ending	Primary sensory ending
(Portion arising from nuclear bag intrafusal fiber)	(Portion arising from nuclear chain intrafusal fiber)
Group Ia afferent[1] fiber	Group Ia afferent[1] fiber
	Group II afferent fiber
Phasic alpha motoneuron	Tonic alpha motoneuron

[1] Group Ia afferent fiber transmits both dynamic and static impulses from primary endings.

Modified from Dubo, H.I.C., and R.C. Darling. 1971. *In* J.A. Downey and R.C. Darling (eds.), Physiological Basis of Rehabilitation Medicine, W.B. Saunders Co., Philadelphia.

The anterior horn cell pool of motor neurons at each segmental level is composed of varying diameters (4-135μ) of alpha and gamma cells. The larger the cells, the more intrafusal or extrafusal fibers they innervate and the faster the conduction time. McPhedran, Wuerker, and Henneman (*34*) reported experimental evidence to prove that the diameter of the motor nerve fiber is related to the number of muscle fibers it supplies. Eccles and Sherrington (*13*) determined the average tension developed by a single motor unit in a given muscle by dividing the total number of motor units in the muscle (determined by counting the number of fibers in a motor nerve before branching) into the amount of tension developed in the total muscle when the nerve was stimulated maximally. In the same paper, an experiment was described in which ventral roots of the spinal cord of a cat were cut, so that only a few intact fibers remained. Then by tapping the tendon and varying the strength of the tapping, it was possible to produce a graded response in normal tendon reflexes.

When 2.5 g of muscle tension resulted from a tendon tap, a single diphasic electrical response occurred. With a 4 g stimulus, a double action potential was produced. They concluded that a 2.5 g response was the average twitch of a single motor unit in the cat. As more and more tension is needed in muscle, small, intermediate, and large motor units are recruited. In other words, the excitability of motor units is determined by the size of the cell body and this size controls recruitment order. Henneman et al. (*21*) state flatly that the recruitment order is always the same, that is, the smaller units are fired first rather than the larger. On the other hand, the inhibition of the motor neurons is the direct opposite, the larger neurons being the most easily inhibited. Basmajian and others have shown that man can be trained to alter the recruitment order with proper training utilizing biofeedback in the form of auditory and visual clues.

Having now established a complex pool of neurons in the anterior gray horn of the spinal cord and in certain cranial nerve nuclei, let us look more closely at the effector cell internal organization in the spinal cord.

ORGANIZATION OF THE MOTOR NEURONAL POOL

A somatotopic distribution of motor neurons in the anterior horn gray matter has been known for some time. The anterior horn cells are broken down into two distinct groups of cells, a medial cell column and a lateral cell column. The medial cell column sends axons out to innervate the proximal muscles of the neck, back, thorax, and pelvis. These motor units form the dorsal ramus of a spinal nerve. The lateral cell column innervates the distal musculature of the limbs and forms the ventral ramus and plexuses of spinal nerves (Figure 5). This motor neuronal pool arrangement is consistent with the belief that there are two systems for motor control: one to control the proximally located axial muscles (particularly

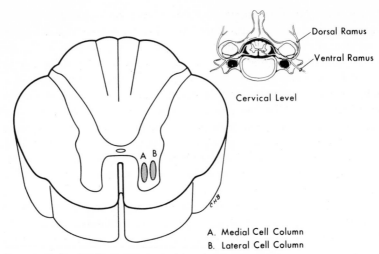

A. Medial Cell Column
B. Lateral Cell Column

Figure 5. Cross section of the spinal cord showing the arrangement of the medial and lateral cell columns in the anterior gray horn.

the extensors) and a second system for control of the distally situated muscles responsible for limb motions (mainly the flexors) (*42*).

SUPRASEGMENTAL CONTROL
OF THE ANTERIOR HORN CELL POOLS (ALPHA CELLS)

Suprasegmental structures, namely any part of the neural axis (neuroaxis) located above the spinal cord, are responsible for governing the output of the motor neurons in the anterior gray horn of the spinal cord. The major descending tracts from suprasegmental areas, beginning at the highest level, are: corticospinal (pyramidal), frontopontine, rubrospinal, reticulospinal, MLF (medial longitudinal fasciculus), and vestibulospinal. Kuypers (*29*) and Lawrence and Kuypers (*30*) were able to show that, by histological examination of previously placed lesions in cats and monkeys, the medial cell column of the anterior horn gray matter received its suprasegmental influences via the reticulospinal, MLF, and vestibulospinal tracts (Figure 6). These selective brain stem lesions affected chiefly the axial muscles and posture maintenance extension groups. Further studies indicated that the lateral cell column in the anterior gray matter received its suprasegmental innervation via the corticospinal, rubrospinal, and reticulospinal tracts (Figure 7) and lesions of these tracts were characterized by the loss of distal muscle control in the extremities.

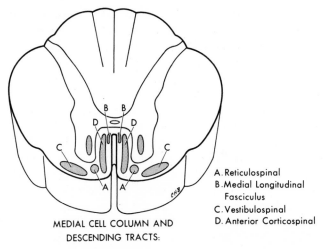

MEDIAL CELL COLUMN AND
DESCENDING TRACTS:

A. Reticulospinal
B. Medial Longitudinal
Fasciculus
C. Vestibulospinal
D. Anterior Corticospinal

Figure 6. The location of suprasegmental pathways that influence the medial cell column of the anterior horn gray matter.

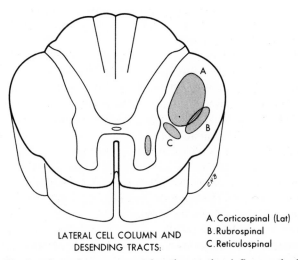

LATERAL CELL COLUMN AND
DESENDING TRACTS:

A. Corticospinal (Lat)
B. Rubrospinal
C. Reticulospinal

Figure 7. The location of suprasegmental pathways that influence the lateral cell column of the anterior horn gray matter.

This distinct division would tend to suggest that the medial cell column does not receive any direct innervation via the corticospinal system. At this time it should be pointed out that the corticospinal tracts, during their descent through the brain stem, decussate in the caudal half of the medulla. In this motor decussation, 85% of the fibers cross in the medulla, forming the lateral corticospinal tract (lateral because it travels in the lateral funiculus of the spinal cord), while the remaining 15% form the anterior corticospinal tract that is uncrossed in the medulla and is found in the anterior funiculus of the spinal cord. The cerebral hemispheres control and receive information from the contralateral side of the body. Therefore, the anterior corticospinal pathways cross but at the segment of the spinal cord where they are going to synapse on the anterior horn cell pool. The lateral corticospinal tracts synapse on the lateral cell column; the anterior corticospinal tracts synapse on the medial cell column neuronal pools (Figure 6).

The larger number of fibers in the lateral corticospinal tracts correlates nicely with the lower innervation ratios necessary to produce fine discrete motor control. In the cat, the pyramidal tract system synapses in the interneuronal pool before connecting to the respective cell column. In monkeys and man (7, 22, 24), monosynaptic connections are present and located primarily in the lateral cell column. Approximately 95% of the corticospinal fiber tracts are multisynaptic while only 5% are monosynaptic. Therefore, a fast pathway to anterior horn cells is available but the major portion of descending pathway is multisynaptic with intercalated neurons in the intermediate gray matter.

From an evolutionary point of view of the process of encephalization in man, the corticospinal tracts greatly outnumber the brain stem descending (rubrospinal) pathways, while in the cat, dog, and similar animals the ratio is reversed. This is an example of the relocation of function in man during the process of encephalization, but it must be reiterated that the lower level brain stem structures still play vital roles in motor control. This also explains why man suffers such irreversible damage to the neopallium (cortex) while cats and dogs recover after similar lesions. For example, the greater encephalization of motor control in primates is exhibited markedly in experiments in which the cat's intra-brain is removed cephad to the subthalamus. The cat is able to walk quite well, yet the primate exhibits poor ability to ambulate even after longer periods following surgery, and seldom regains fine precision skills with the hand (2, 12). This can be related to the increase in size of the tracts descending from the cortex in primates. The disagreement that still exists in the literature in relation to experimental lesions is due to differences in species used in experiments, the recovery time after surgery, and the location of the lesions.

ASCENDING PATHWAYS: THE FEEDBACK SYSTEM

The effective activation of our "little motors," with which we are so greatly endowed, for purposeful movement depends heavily on the input of information to the central nervous system from the great number of receptors scattered throughout the biological system.

C.S. Sherrington (*39*) classified cell receptors into three special classes that are not entirely exclusive, but rather are classified according to where the stimuli are located:

1. *Exteroceptive sensations* (germ layer of development ectoderm): environmental changes on the surface of the body such as touch, pressure, pain, and temperature.
2. *Proprioceptive sensations* (germ layer of development of mesoderm): changes of the body itself (inside, deep) as in inner ear, muscles, tendons, ligaments, and joints.
3. *Interoceptive sensations* (germ layer of development entoderm): stimuli within the body primarily from the internal organs, as in the circulatory, digestive, and secretory systems.

Smell, vision, and hearing were included among receptors as a special category because they provided information about events and objects at a distance from the body and are designated as "teloreceptors."

Still others, e.g., Willis and Grossman (*44*), classify receptors under four major areas:

> Special—vision, audition, taste, olfaction, and vestibular
> Superficial—touch, pressure, pain, and temperature
> Deep—position, vibration, deep press, deep pain
> Visceral—hunger, nausea, visceral pain

Because we are focusing our attention on the control of skeletal muscle, our discussion is centered upon general somatic sensations. More specifically, it might be asked what receptor mechanisms are involved in the carrying out of purposeful skeletal muscle contraction. Before exploring this question, it should be recalled that it was earlier speculated that there existed a duality of both the alpha and gamma motor units within the anterior horn pools. This duality would tend to point towards a dual sensory feedback mechanism. From the previous description of sensation (by Sherrington), we can divide general somatic sensations into two major categories, proprioceptive and exteroceptive.

Proprioceptive information is concerned with the orientation of the head and body in space, the angle of joints, and the degree of shortening in skeletal muscle. Exteroception sensation is concerned with the effects of the environment on the body, either by direct contact or distal stimuli (e.g., pain, temperature, touch, pressure, olfactory, visual, and auditory changes). The latter receptors are generally referred to as special somatic sensation (i.e., teloreceptors).

Looking even more closely at the monitoring systems related to skeletal muscle, it is easier to discuss this sensory feedback system by dividing the receptors into those found directly within skeletal muscle tissue or nearby (intrinsic feedback system), and those receptor mechanisms located outside skeletal muscle proper, thus comprising the extrinsic feedback system (e.g., ligaments, joint capsules, skin).

Intrinsic Feedback System

There are three types of receptors that make up the intrinsic monitoring system of skeletal muscle (*33*). These receptors are, as presented in Figure 8:

> 1. Muscle spindle
> 2. Tendon organ
> 3. Vater-Pacinian Corpuscles

Muscle Spindle

The muscle spindle is the most elaborately structured of the intrinsic receptors. This receptor appears to be found in all muscles responsible for movement, including many muscles supplied by motor cranial nerves. It is important to note that the density of muscle spindles is different in the various muscles of the body according to cross-sectional area and location. For example, in man's abductor pollicis brevis muscle there are 80 spindles (*38*), while in the massive latissimus dorsi muscle there are 368 (*43*). By estimating the number of spindles per gram of muscle tissue, the values of 29.3 for the abductor muscle and 1.4 for the latissimus dorsi are obtained. These factors show that muscles responsible for fine precision movement have more spindles per gram of tissue than those muscles used in gross patterns of movements.

The muscle spindle must be viewed by its components in order to comprehend the relationship between its anatomical structure and its physiological role. The principle aspects of a spindle's anatomy are: a

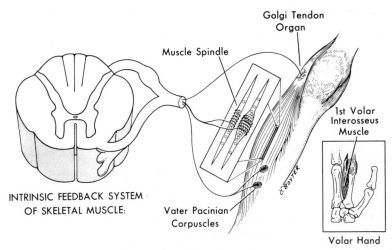

Figure 8. Schematic drawing of the receptors that make up the intrinsic monitoring system of skeletal muscle.

spindle-shaped connective tissue capsule filled with fluid, and the intrafusal muscle fibers. Intrafusal muscle fibers in man average approximately 10/spindle. The intrafusal fibers are attached at both ends of the spindle capsule and hence arranged parallel to the extrafusal muscle fibers. Most spindles contain two distinct types of intrafusal muscle fibers with different diameters. They are named according to the arrangement of their nuclei into thick fibers called "nuclear bag fibers" and thinner fibers termed "nuclear chain fibers," as in Figure 4.

Further study of the spindle innervation has revealed that: (a) the primary sensory (annulospiral) endings (Ia or Group I afferents) are related to both intrafusal muscle fibers, and (b) the secondary sensory (flower spray) endings (IIa or Group II afferents) appear to be present chiefly on the nuclear chain fibers, but this is not always true. These two intrinsic receptor components of the spindle are related to the length-control system (i.e., they function to monitor length and velocity of the muscles).

Tendon Organ

The tendon organs are less complex in structure than the muscle spindles. The tendon organ is composed of a large myelinated group of nerve fibers that terminate with branching of fine endings between the bundles of collagenous fibers of a tendon (see Figure 8). These finely branched nerve fibers are surrounded by a connective tissue capsule. In order to understand their function it is important to note that, in contrast to muscle spindles, the tendon organs are arranged in series with the extrafusal muscle fibers. This means that whether the muscle is actively shortened or stretched, the tendon organs are going to be stimulated. The tendon organs are, therefore, responsible for recording tension changes in muscles.

In regard to number, Swett and Eldred (40) reported that in certain muscles the number of tendon organs is only slightly below the number of muscle spindles. It appears that the tendon organ may be of greater importance in motor control than previously thought.

Vater-Pacinian Corpuscles (Pacinian Bodies)

The Pacinian corpuscles are the most widely distributed and the largest of the encapsulated receptors. They are each supplied by a large myelinated fiber and differ from the other encapsulated organs mainly in the more elaborate development of their perineural capsule. The capsule is formed by a large number of concentric lamellae whose outer rings are composed of a single continuous layer of flattened cells supported by collagen fibrils (Figure 4).

The entire length of the unmyelinated fiber within the capsule is sensitive to deformation. In terms of function, the Pacinian corpuscles have in the course of time been assumed to be receptors for pressure. Since these receptors are large, supplied by a single nerve fiber, and easy to locate, they have proved useful and popular for study.

Various studies have shown that, under steady pressure, the corpuscles respond with a rapidly adapting discharge (20). If, however, they are stimulated rhythmically with a vibratory stimulus, the action potentials recorded from the large myelinated afferent fibers follow the stimulus frequency from 50–800 cycles/sec (25). It appears that the Pacinian corpuscles in muscle send, in response to vibration and pressure, additional information to the CNS concerning the contractile state of the muscle and contribute to the reflex control of movement.

EFFERENT INNERVATION OF THE MUSCLE

As mentioned earlier, it has been shown that most spindles contain two types of intrafusal fibers, and further studies have shown that there is more than one type of gamma fiber innervating the intrafusal fibers. Two gamma fibers were differentiated by the difference in their terminal endings. One ending is represented by motor end plates similar to those found in extrafusal muscle fibers (the myoneural junctions).

The other terminal endings form a diffuse collection of fine axonal fibers in the net-like arrangement (Figure 4). Barker (4) referred to them as plate endings and trail endings. Whether they can be correlated with what Boyd (8) called α_1 and α_2 is still to be resolved. It is also still disputed whether the plate endings occur only on nuclear bag fibers and whether trail endings occur exclusively on chain fibers.

To add even more complexity to the efferent fiber innervation is the report by Adal and Barker (1), demonstrating that nerve fibers supplying extrafusal muscle fibers also send branches to intrafusal muscle fibers, sometimes referred to as beta fibers or slow alpha fibers.

The complexity of the muscle spindle structure, innervation, and variation leaves many unanswered questions to be investigated. However, it can be stated that the spindles inform the central nervous system of two important forms of information, muscle length and speed of stretching, both of which are essential for the activity of spinal reflexes and for muscle control by supra-segmental centers such as the cerebellum.

ACTIVATION OF EXTRAFUSAL MUSCLE FIBERS

In the resting state, normal muscle can be palpated and it will be observed that there is a certain level of tension. This normal resting tension is referred to as muscle tone. There is much controversy regarding the explanation of muscle tone. It is clear, however, that muscle tone is due to reflex responses from the intrinsic receptors of muscle. Sherrington demonstrated this fact when he experimentally cut the extrinsic afferent fibers leaving only the intrinsic afferent fibers intact, and the tone was not changed. It was later found that this tone was due to the muscle spindle receptors and is referred to as reflex tone. Thus the spindles are responsible for regulating muscle tone through tonic stretch reflexes.

In the activation of purposeful movement, the gamma innervation is important in setting the tone of the muscles to be used. That is, increased gamma activity will set the spindle at a more active level and thereby reflexly increase the tone of the extrafusal muscle fibers, as well as contribute to their control. The alpha motor neurons, on the other hand, are responsible for the contraction of the extrafusal fibers.

The integrative function of gamma and alpha motor neurons in the initiation and execution of purposeful movements has been the subject of many studies. It still remains to be clarified as to what system is responsible for the initiation, activation, and completion of movement.

Granit, Holmgren, and Merton (18) suggested that the brain can produce movements from two possible routes: (a) pathways acting on alpha cells, and (b) pathways acting on gamma cells (which then act on alpha cells via afferent fiber connections).

The direct alpha controlling system (motor unit) has the advantage of avoiding the time delay necessary to activate the intrafusal fiber to spindles, intrinsic receptor, and finally the alpha motor neuron pool. It is believed that the alpha and gamma motor units are co-activated, thereby allowing a more efficient use of the intrinsic feedback system, thus giving better control of muscle contraction (i.e., length, force, and velocity), in both antagonistic and agonistic muscle groups during most activities of daily living. The fast route for direct alpha motor neuron activation is to initiate movement, while the gamma motor neurons indirect route of alpha recruitment is used to assure the suprasegmental centers that the proper alpha cell activation is being facilitated to perform the desired skeletal muscle task. We can then understand why the intrinsic receptor feedback system is a servo-mechanism to CNS activation.

Extrinsic Feedback System

Attention can now be directed to the extrinsic receptor system, i.e., those receptors located outside of skeletal muscle proper. Specifically, we are concerned with joint capsules, ligaments, skin, and subcutaneous tissues (Figure 9).

Ligaments and joint capsules provide a precise monitoring system in terms of the joint angle, speed, and direction of joint mobility. Each joint angle elicits a steady discharge, the frequency of which varies according to angular displacement. The frequency signal, which indicates positioning, also specifies the length of the muscles that cross that joint. However, extrinsic receptors are generally divided into two major categories: cutaneous receptors and joint receptors. Cutaneous receptors are further divided into mechanoreceptors, thermoreceptors, and pain receptors.

Cutaneous Receptors

Mechanoreceptors There are several different kinds of mechanoreceptors: hair plexus, Merkel's disc, and Meissner's corpuscles. These three receptors all respond to tactile stimuli. It also appears that free nerve endings may be included in this group.

Thermoreceptors The sensations of warm and cold have been linked to Ruffini corpuscles and Krause's end bulbs, respectively. However, areas of the body where neither receptors are found also respond to temperature changes. It appears that an adequate stimulus is all that is needed and not the absolute temperature to elicit a discharge in temperature sensitive fibers. Hensel, Iggo, and Witt (*23*) reported that the temperature range for maximum discharge is between 38–42°C for the warm fibers and 16–27°C for the cold fibers.

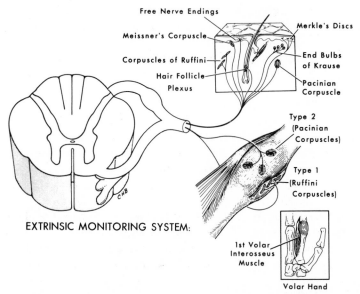

Figure 9. Schematic drawing of receptors that make up the extrinsic monitoring system of skeletal muscle.

Pain receptors It is generally accepted that the free fine-nerve endings in the skin and other organs are responsible for pain reception. There also appears to be further agreement that the sensation of pain is mediated by two groups of fibers: thinly myelinated ones for fast pain and unmyelinated fibers for slow pain. In spite of a great deal of clinical interest and study, little is definitely clear at this time and the complexity of pain reception continues to leave many questions unanswered.

Special attention must be given to Pacinian corpuscles because, for a long period of time, these receptors, located in the subcutaneous tissue as well as other places, have been assumed to be receptors for a variety of stimuli. It now appears that these receptors in the skin are responsible for recording vibrations. The functional importance is still not clear and there remain many unanswered questions.

Joint Receptors It is a well-known and appreciated fact that we are able to recognize very small movements in joints. Yet, if the joint capsule is anesthetized and one's eyes are closed, it is no longer possible to monitor joint positions. Recent investigations by Freeman and Wyke (*17*) have shown that, although the receptors in joints have structures similar to those in other tissues (e.g., Ruffini endings, Pacinian corpuscles, etc.)

it is advisable to avoid these analogies. The above authors have grouped joint reception into four categories based on their functional properties. The following is a brief description of the four receptor types:

Type I Receptors   These endings have been linked to Ruffini endings, having an ovoid corpuscle with a thin connective tissue capsule. These receptors occur in fibrous joint capsules and a few in the extrinsic ligaments. The changing frequency of the impulses from these receptors signals the direction of movement and also the speed.

Type II Receptors   These endings have a single terminal within a thick laminated capsule with a more heavily myelinated fiber than Type I receptors. They resemble Pacinian corpuscles. They occur only in fibrous joint capsules and are sensitive to rapid movements and are thus called acceleration receptors.

Type III Receptors   This type of receptor is the largest of the joint receptors. They resemble Golgi tendon organs in structure and only occur in the ligaments within the outside of joint capsules. They appear to record the position of joints having a high threshold and a slow adaptability.

Type IV Receptors   This type of receptor is made up of fine branching unmyelinated fibers that are located in the fibrous joint capsule, joint ligaments, synovial capsules, and fat pads. They primarily are interpreted to be the pain receptors related to joints and their immediate tissues.

Attempts to relate sensory receptor structure and location to function are not justifiable at this time because they are too poorly understood. The type of receptor can be determined by its ability to adapt to a constant stimulus. Those showing a great amount of adaptation have a phasic function, those showing a slow amount of adaptation have a tonic function. At this time it is clear that the intrinsic annulospiral endings (IA) respond to adequate stimuli of muscle length, tendon organs for tension and Pacinian corpuscles for pressure. Similar relationships for cutaneous and subcutaneous receptors are not yet so clearly defined.

The use of various stimulating techniques to elicit cutaneous receptor responses in physical therapy by brushing, tapping, rubbing, and temperature variation certainly indicates an area of uncharted research. Indeed, a basic understanding of our external monitoring system, which is so vital to the orientation of man to his immediate environment, is extremely complex, as indicated by the number of receptors and receptor subtypes (e.g., bare nerve endings, Merkel's disks, Meissner's corpuscles, hair follicle receptors, Pacinian bodies, etc.). It must be remembered that, in order for man to have adequate protection from harmful injuries, the external receptor system must not be classified as a secondary feedback system in analyzing the activation of skeletal muscle for purposeful movements because, without such a cutaneous sensory feedback system, the survival of mankind and individual lower phylums would be greatly in doubt.

Sensory feedback plays a vital role in an effective, motor-operating biological machine, a factor clearly seen in experiments with dorsal root transection that abolishes all ordinary use of a differentiated limb. Such an extremity hangs limply as if paralyzed until a recovery period has transpired, when other systems then substitute for the sensory damaged receptors (e.g., vision for proprioception deficits in the limbs).

MOTOR AND SENSORY DEFICITS—
THEIR EFFECTS ON MOTOR CONTROL

Segmental Deficits

Motor Unit Lesions (alpha cells) Infections, injuries, or surgical interruption of any part of an alpha motor unit will result in a complete loss of the functional capacity of that motor unit. Figure 10 illustrates the various sites at which motor units are affected. When motor neurons or the motor axon are damaged (sites #1 and #2) a lower motor neuron lesion is present (e.g., poliomyelitis or damage to either ventral or dorsal ramus). Such a motor deficit is characterized by loss of voluntary and reflex contractions of the muscle fibers supplied by that motor neuron, which causes muscles to be flaccid. The muscle fibers begin to show signs of atrophy in as little

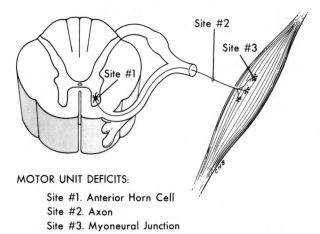

MOTOR UNIT DEFICITS:
   Site #1. Anterior Horn Cell
   Site #2. Axon
   Site #3. Myoneural Junction

Figure 10. Schematic diagram illustrating the various alpha motor units deficit sites. *Site 1,* lower motor neuron lesion; *Site 2,* motor peripheral nerve deficit; *Site 3,* myoneural junction deficit.

as 7–10 days. The longer the duration, the more conspicuous this becomes. The synaptic vesicles within axon terminals at the myoneural junction (in Site #3) are believed to be the sites for storage of acetylcholine (ACh). When a nerve impulse arrives at the presynaptic membrane. ACh is released into the synaptic gutter and stimulates receptor sites on the post-synaptic membrane. This activity increases the permeability of the sarcolemmal membrane of the muscle fiber and, in turn, causes depolarization and a muscle contraction.

If for any reason an inadequate amount of ACh is secreted, the muscles involved are susceptible to fatigue. Clinically, myesthenia gravis exhibits this type of symptom and is treated by medication that allows a preservation of ACh at the end-plate terminals for longer periods of time.

Sensory Unit Lesions   As far back as 1895, Sherrington demonstrated that complete differentiation of an extremity resulted in paralysis of the limb (Site #1, Figure 11). This is referred to as a dorsal rhizotomy and is used clinically as a treatment for the relief of severe spasticity in spinal cord injured patients. Taub and Berman *(41)*, however, have shown that conditioned movements are retained by the animals given time to recover. This led the author to propose an intrinsic CNS feedback system. It is interesting to observe the results of cutting intrinsic sensory units of a muscle (Site #2, Figure 11) while leaving the extrinsic sensory units intact. Under such conditions little impairment of function is noticeable. However, if the extrinsic sensory units are sectioned (Site #3, Figure 11) thus leaving the intrinsic sensory units intact, the muscle is rendered useless immediately after surgery and for several days to weeks. Then, return of function is observed but never to the same speed or previous skill.

It can be concluded that, of the two sensory unit systems in the highest forms of encephalization, the extrinsic sensory units are necessary for the conscious control of skeletal muscle activity in the execution of purposeful movement during highly skilled activity of daily living. Yet, given time, the plasticity of the CNS and perhaps its CNS intrinsic feedback system can overcome the peripheral nervous system's sensory deficit.

Suprasegmental Deficits

Motor units of the spinal cord and brain stem are under the control of segmental sensory units, inter-neuron ascending tracts, and inter-neuron descending tracts. The controlling mechanisms of motor units are extremely complex because all systems mentioned above play on them continuously. It is still not possible at this time to give precise answers to questions regarding suprasegmental control of skeletal muscle activity.

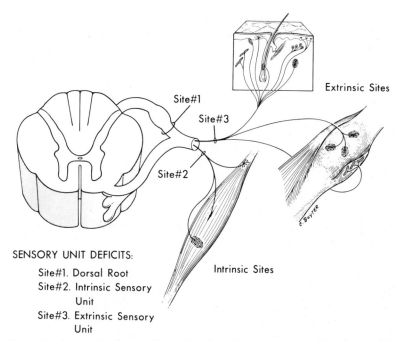

SENSORY UNIT DEFICITS:

   Site#1. Dorsal Root
   Site#2. Intrinsic Sensory
       Unit
   Site#3. Extrinsic Sensory
       Unit

Figure 11. Schematic diagram illustrating the various sensory unit deficit sites. *Site 1,* combined sensory deficit; *Site 2,* intrinsic sensory deficit; *Site 3,* extrinsic sensory deficit.

However, clinical and laboratory experimentation has given some general verification of the neuroaxis controlling centers.

In man, the descending tracts (corticospinal, corticopontine, cortico-bulbar, and other corticofugal tracts) to the spinal cord and brain stem are responsible for the conscious control of purposeful motor activity. Lesions affecting this suprasegmental controlling system are twofold: first, those affecting the corticospinal or corticobulbar system, and second, those affecting other suprasegmental structures (e.g., basal ganglia, cerebellum, and brain stem).

Thus, there are four suprasegmental controlling centers for skeletal muscle activity. The first center is the telencephalon (cerebral cortex). The cortex sends descending tracts (corticobulbar, corticofugal, and cortico-spinal) to the brain stem motor nuclei and the anterior horn cells of the spinal cord.These descending tracts mediate any voluntary movement and, as was mentioned earlier, the spinal system is further subdivided into medial and lateral descending tracts. Lesions affecting this system produce in general what is known clinically as an upper motor neuron lesion. Such a motor deficit is characterized by the loss of voluntary control of muscular activity, hyperreflexia, hypertonus, and disuse atrophy. In the adult man, the site of the lesion produces varying results and even varies from person to person. Thus, it is clinically difficult to locate precisely the site of the deficit without some further diagnostic tests, for example the brain scan.

Cerebral Cortex Effects of ablations of the primary motor cortex produce a paralysis of the contralateral skeletal muscles. The distally located limb muscles are more seriously affected than the proximally located muscles because of their greater cerebral representation. The recovery of function varies greatly and depends on the size of the lesion and the age of the individual.

Descending Cortico Tracts Lesions affecting the descending tracts at different levels of the neuraxis also vary greatly from species to species, from person to person, and from lesion site to lesion site (e.g., internal capsule lesions versus pyramidal tract lesions, upper brain stem versus lower brain stem). Internal capsule lesions are much more damaging than lesions of the corticospinal tract in the brain stem because the corticospinal system is only one tract that mediates voluntary movement, while lesions in the internal capsule affect a greater number of descending tracts (i.e., corticobulbar, corticopontine, corticorubro, etc.).

Basal Ganglia Although experimental approaches to studying the function of the basal ganglia have not proven to be satisfactory and in most cases have led to confusion, the functions of the basal ganglia and their deficits are provided by clinical information from the signs and symptoms that are produced by diseases affecting these structures. Because we are addressing our discussion to motor control, we are focusing on the motor effects of basal ganglia diseases.

All the diseases of the basal ganglia are characterized by disturbances of motility.

Akinesia The patient has difficulty in initiating and carrying out voluntary movements.

Dystonia Most frequently an increase in tone is seen and it is found in opposing muscles. It is called rigidity. This rigidity is different from spasticity in that it is constant at all positions of the extremity. Certain diseases of the basal ganglia also produce a reduction in muscle tone. In these cases, the limbs are usually lacking tone in both agonistic and antagonistic muscle groups.

Involuntary Movements Disarrangement of the basal ganglia circulatory or related structures may permit abnormal activity of the cortical motor mechanisms and hence produce the following clinical manifestations of involuntary movements:

Chorea—spontaneous abrupt and rapid successive movements involving the extremities and the face.

Parkinsonism—muscle rigidity and tremor resulting in disturbances of posture and the ease and execution of rapidity of voluntary movements.

Ballismus—wild flinging, twisting and rolling, and involuntary movements.

More precise information is needed to establish the function of the basal ganglia. Present neurophysiological techniques have provided no meaningful understanding and more refined and specialized techniques will have to be perfected to explore the relationship between the basal ganglia and complex motor activities.

Cerebellum   There are three major functional components that may be related to anatomical lesions of the cerebellum:

1. coordination of somatic motor activity
2. regulation of muscle tone
3. regulation of mechanisms that influence and maintain equilibrium

The cerebellum is divided developmentally into three parts:

Archicerebellum—the oldest part of the cerebellum, formed by sensory input from the vestibular apparatus. This sensory input forms the floccular-nodular lobe of the cerebellum.

Palaeocerebellum—the anterior lobe of the cerebellum, linked with the input of information from the spinal cord (e.g., muscles, joints, ligaments, etc.).

Neocerebellum—the posterior lobe of the cerebellum develops parallel with the development of the neocortex from which it receives its major input.

Cerebellar Lesions

Archicerebellar syndrome results in the loss of equilibrium without the loss of voluntary movements. The clinical signs are ataxia of trunk muscles leading to a tendency to fall backwards, to sway from side to side, and to walk with a wide base of support.

Palaeocerebellar syndrome results in severe disturbances in posture and increased extensor muscle tone.

Neocerebellar syndrome results primarily in the loss of isolated finer movements of the extremities.

It must be noted that the clinical evidence that is available is vague, inconsistant, and conflicting with the results obtained from animal experiments.

Brain Stem   The brain stem anatomically consists of the dorsal thalamus, midbrain, pons, and medulla. It is composed of groups of nerve cells and fibers running to and from the cerebral cortex, cerebellum, brain stem, spinal cord, and other related nuclei centers.

In between these groups of nuclei and fibers are cells of a specialized type that in most areas are loosely arranged but interconnected by synapses. This cellular arrangement produces a net-like appearance; hence it was named the reticular formation (RF). In the process of evolution, the reticular formation underwent specific development in conjunction with other neural structures.

The reticular formation is in such a strategic position in the brain stem that it receives data from almost all tracts passing through it and in turn has connections with all levels of the neuroaxis.

Histologically, there are specific areas of the RF present in each level of the brain stem. It is convenient to speak of the reticular system as comprising three regions or nuclear groups (5). Group 1 consists of the lateral and paramedian nuclei of the medulla, both projecting to the cerebellum. Group 2 consists of the parvicellular nuclei of the medulla and pons, sending fibers to the medial part of the reticular formation. Group 3 is composed of nuclei (magnocellular) in the medial medulla, pons, and midbrain; these nuclei receive afferents from the lateral or sensory part of the RF (parvicellular nuclei) Group 2. Group 3 sends fibers longitudinally in the brain stem, giving collaterals off to other reticular cells. These collateral connections make possible the wide-spread polysynaptic connections of the RF throughout the entire CNS.

Functional Aspects There are numerous functions known to be related to RF efferent connections. However, because we are addressing ourselves to motor control we are limiting our coverage to its effects on alpha and gamma cells. It must be pointed out that the RF appears to be important to almost all functions related to nervous system control. For example, Scheibel and Scheibel (37) found that in addition to connecting with the spinal cord, the thalamus, and other brain stem areas, collaterals extend from ascending and descending tracts of the RF to all cranial nerve nuclei.

Magoun and Rhines (32) showed that electrical stimulation of the RF could alter motor activity in the spinal cord. Later Rossi and Zanchetti (36) showed more specifically that both alpha and gamma motor neurons can be facilitated or inhibited from the brain stem reticular formation. Stimulation of the medullary reticulospinal projection area causes inhibition of the spinal cord alpha cells. This effect is further illustrated by the fact that decerebrate rigidity is suppressed by stimulation of the medullary reticulospinal projection system. It is quite evident that reticospinal pathways are capable of acting on gamma cells as well. It has as yet to be determined whether the medullary reticular area has excitatory or inhibitory effects as it could well have both.

The complexity of the effects on gamma cells has been well pointed out by Lindbloom and Ottosson (*31*), who reported that reflex activity can be inhibited and facilitated from the same brain stem area.

From the literature pertaining to the effect of the RF on the spinal cord, it appears that the inhibitory area of the medulla is the site of origin of the inhibitory reticulospinal tract. While the area of facilitation appears to encompass much broader areas, including the pontine RF, it seems at this time that the inhibitory pathways to the cord are direct. Facilatory effects must occur by fibers originating in other suprasegmental areas that terminate in reticulospinal neurons in the reticular formation of the brain stem.

It is interesting to speculate, as was done with the corticospinal tracts, that there exist two major descending reticulospinal pathways; one from the medulla (lateral) the other from the pons (medial), based upon the termination sites as reported by Nyberg-Hansen (*35*). It is not possible, however, to speculate what their effects are on the anterior horn motor pool. It appears that the effects the reticular formation pathways have on the spinal cord depend chiefly on the properties of the spinal cord. Therefore, other suprasegmental structures (vestibular nuclei, red nucleus, superior colliculus, the cerebellum, and the cerebral cortex) must work cooperatively with the reticular formation to bring about modifications in motor activity.

With the continued improvement of neurophysiological research techniques involving single cell recording and fiber recordings and the correlation of data from clinical case histories, it may be possible to explain the disorders of motor functions that occur from disease processes. The introduction of the use of scanning techniques to view the body is especially intriguing as it opens a whole new era of CNS exploration.

LITERATURE CITED

1. Adal, M.N., and D. Barker. 1965. Intramuscular branching of fusimotor fibers. J. Physiol. (Lond.) 177:288–299.
2. Bard, P., and D. McK. Rioch. 1937. A study of four cats deprived of neocortex and additional portions of the forebrain. Bull. Johns Hopkins Hospital 60:73.
3. Barker, D. 1962. The structure and distribution of muscle receptors. *In* D. Barker (ed.), Symposium on Muscle Receptors. pp. 227–240. Hong Kong University Press; Oxford University Press, London.
4. Barker, D. 1966. The motor innervation of the muscle spindle. *In* R.

Granit (ed.), Noble Symposium I: Muscular Afferents and Motor Control. pp. 51–58. Olmgvist A. Wiksell, Stockholm; John Wiley and Sons, New York.

5. Barr, M.L. 1974. The Human Nervous System, 2nd Ed. Harper and Row, New York.

6. Basmajian, J.V. 1963. Control and training of individual motor units. Science 141:440–441.

7. Bernhard, C.G., E. Bohm, and I. Petersen. 1953. Investigations on the organization of the corticospinal system in monkeys. Acta Physiol. Scand. 29, (Suppl.) 106:79.

8. Boyd, I.A. 1962. The structure and innervation of nuclear bag muscle fiber system and the nuclear chain muscle fiber system in mammalian muscle spindles. Philos. Trans. R. Soc. Lond. (Biol. Sci.) 245:81.

9. Brodal, A. 1969. Neurological Anatomy, 2nd Ed. Oxford University Press, London.

10. Clark, D.A. 1931. Muscle counts of motor units: a study in innervation ratios. Am. J. Physiol. 96:296.

11. Cooper, S., and P.M. Daniels. 1963. Muscle spindles in man; their morphology in the lumbricals and the deep muscles of the neck. Brain 86:563–586.

12. Denny-Brown, D. 1966. The cerebral control of movement. Liverpool University Press, Liverpool.

13. Eccles, J.C., and C.S. Sherrington. 1930. Numbers and contraction–values of individual motor units examined in some muscles of the limb. Proc. R. Soc. Lond. (Biol.) 106:326–357.

14. Evarts, E.V. 1966. Pyramidal tract activity associated with a conditioned hand movement in the monkey. J. Neurophysiol. 29: 1011–1027.

15. Evarts, E.V. 1971. Activity of thalamic and cortical neurons in relation to learned movement in the monkey. Int. J. Neurol. 8: 321–326.

16. Evarts, E.V. 1973. Brain mechanisms in movement. Sci. Am. 229: 96–103.

17. Freeman, M.A.F., and B. Wyke. 1967. The innervation of the knee joint, an anatomical and histological study in the cat. J. Anat. 101:505–532.

18. Granit, R., B. Holmgren, and P.A. Merton. 1955. The two routes for excitation of muscle and their subservience to the cerebellum. J. Physiol. (Lond.) 130:213–224.

19. Grant, J.C., and J.V. Basmajian. 1965. Grant's method of anatomy, 7th Ed. Williams and Wilkins Co., Baltimore.

20. Gray, J.A.B., and P.B.C. Matthews. 1951. Response of pacinian corpuscles in the cat's toe. J. Physiol. (Lond.) 113:475–482.

21. Henneman, E., G. Somjim, and D.O. Carpenter. 1965. Functional significance of cell size in spinal motorneurons. J. Neurophysiol. 28:560.

22. Henneman, E. 1974. Motor functions of cerebral cortex. In V.B. Mountcastle (ed.), Medical Physiology. Vol. 1, 748–749. The C.V. Mosby Company, St. Louis.

23. Hensel, H.A., A. Iggo, and I. Witt. 1960. Quantitative study of sensitive cutaneous thermoreceptors with C afferent fibers. J. Physiol. (Lond.) 153:113–126.
24. Hoff, E.C., and H.E. Hoff. 1934. Spinal termination of the projection fibers from the motor cortex of primates. Brain. 57:454–474.
25. Hunt, C.C. 1961. On the nature of vibration receptors in the hind limb of the cat. J. Physiol. (Lond.) 155:175–186.
26. Jasper, H.H. 1958. Recent advances in our understanding of ascending activities of the reticular system. In H.H. Jasper, L.D. Proctor, R.S. Knighton, W.C. Moshay, and R.T. Costello (eds.), Reticular Formation of the Brain. pp. 423–434. Little, Brown and Co. Inc., Boston.
27. Kemp, J.M., and T.P.S. Powell. 1971. The connections of the striatum and the globus pallidus: synthesis and speculation. Philos. Trans. R. Soc. Lond. (Biol. Sci.) 262:441–457.
28. Kennedy, W.R. 1970. Innervation of normal human muscle spindle. Neurology 20:463–475.
29. Kuypers, H.G.J.M. 1963. The organization of the motor system. Int. J. Neurol. 4:78–91.
30. Lawrence, H.G., and J.M. Kuypers. 1965. Pyramidal and non-pyramidal pathways in monkeys. Anatomical and functional correlation. Science 148:973–975.
31. Lindblom, U.F., and J.O. Ottosson. 1956. Bulbar influence on spinal cord dorsum potentials and neutral root reflexes. Acta. Physiol. Scand. 35:203–214.
32. Magoun, H.W., and R. Rhines. 1946. An inhibitory mechanism in the bulbar reticular formation. J. Neurophysiol. 9:165–171.
33. Mathews, P.B.C. 1964. Muscle spindles and their motor control. Physiol. Rev. 44:219.
34. McPhredran, A.M., R.B. Wuerker, and E. Henneman. 1965. Properties of motor units in a homogeneous red muscle (soleus) of the cat. J. Neurophysiol. 28:71–84.
35. Nyberg-Hansen, R. 1965. Sites and mode of termination of reticulo-spinal fibers in the cat. An experimental study with Silver impregnation methods. J. Comp. Neurol. 124:71–100.
36. Rossi, G.F., and A. Zanchetti. 1957. The brain stem reticular formation. Arch. Ital. Biol. 95:199–435.
37. Scheibel, M.E., and A.B. Scheibel. 1958. Structural substrates for integrative patterns in the brain stem reticular core. In H.H. Jasper, L.D. Proctor, R.S. Knighton, W.C. Moshay, and R.T. Costello (eds.), Reticular Formation of the Brain. pp. 31–55. Little, Brown and Co. Inc., Boston.
38. Schulze, M.L. 1955–56. Die absolute and relative Zahl der Muskel-spundeln in dea kurgen. Daumenmuskeln des Menschen. Ant. Anz. 102:290–291.
39. Sherrington, C.S. 1967. The integrative action of the nervous system. Charles Scribner Sons, New York, Reprinted, Yale University Press, New Haven.
40. Swett, J.E., and E. Eldred. 1960. Distribution and numbers of stretch receptors in medial gastrocnemius and soleus muscles of the cat. Anat. Rec. 137:453–460.

41. Taub, E., and Berman, A.J. 1968. Movement and learning in the absence of sensory feedback. *In* S.J. Freedman (ed.), The Neuropsychology of Spatially Oriented Behavior. Dorsey Press, Homewood, Ill.
42. Truex, R.C., and M.B. Carpenter. 1969. Human Neuroanatomy, 6th Ed. Williams and Wilkins Co., Baltimore.
43. Voss, H. 1956. Zahl and Anordnung der Muskelspendeln in den oberen Zungenbeinmuskeln, im. m. trapezious und m. latissimus dorsi. Anat. Anz. 103:443–446.
44. Willis, W.D., and R.C. Grossman. 1973. Medical Neurobiology. The C.V. Mosby Co., Saint Louis.

THE CELLULAR COMPOSITION OF HUMAN SKELETAL MUSCLE

C. David Ianuzzo

CELLULAR CHARACTERISTICS OF MUSCLE FIBER TYPES

The studies of Ranvier in the last century observed mammalian skeletal muscles to be structurally and functionally heterogeneous. Within the past two decades the development of sophisticated physiological, histochemical, and biochemical techniques, along with the invention of the electron microscope, has allowed our understanding of these differences to reach the molecular and ultrastructural levels. It is now firmly established that the cells composing red and white muscles have different morphological, metabolic, and contractile characteristics. Until recently, these techniques were primarily applied to studies using animals other than man, for obvious reasons. Since the development and wide spread use of the muscle biopsy technique, along with methods of microanalysis, studies on man have become increasingly more numerous. Although information concerned with the heterogeneity of human muscle fibers is still meager, the purpose of this chapter is to summarize the ultrastructural, histochemical, biochemical, and contractile characteristics of human muscle fiber types. In addition, a brief summary of selected experimental conditions that alter fiber type character is included. Where data on man are not available, an attempt has been made to extrapolate from animal studies.

Structure of the Muscle Cell

The organizational unit of skeletal muscle is the muscle fiber. The muscle cell is a cylindrically shaped, multinucleated cell covered with a plasma

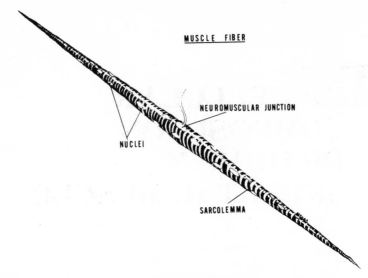

Figure 1. A schematic drawing of a muscle fiber pointing out the striations, multi-nucleation, a single innervation, and the sarcolemma.

membrane (called the sarcolemma), and it usually has but one innervation (Figure 1). The major subcellular division of the muscle fiber is the myofibril, which has a longitudinal orientation and is comprised of repeating units of sarcomeres. The sarcomere is the basic contractile unit of the muscle cell. Its boundaries are defined by heavy dense lines termed Z-lines (Figure 2). Located within the sarcomere are the contractile thin and thick filaments. It is the arrangement of these protein filaments that determines the major banding of the sarcomere (i.e., A and I bands) and the cross-striated appearance of the muscle fiber. The thick myosin filament has cross-bridge projections that extend to the thin actin filaments. Contained within the cross-bridge is the enzyme myosin ATPase, which catalyzes the hydrolysis of ATP during muscle contraction. The ATP utilized for muscle contraction is primarily produced within the mitochondrion. These organelles are located in juxtaposition to the contractile apparatus in the intermyofibrillar space and also in concentrated aggregates beneath the sarcolemma. The muscle cell contains two tubular systems that participate in the events leading to activation of the contractile proteins, i.e., events of excitation-contraction coupling (Figure 2). The transverse tubules (T-tubules) are invaginated continuations of the sarcolemma. This tubular system extends to the inner most parts of the fiber, encircling the myofibril in mammalian muscle at the level of the A-I junction of the

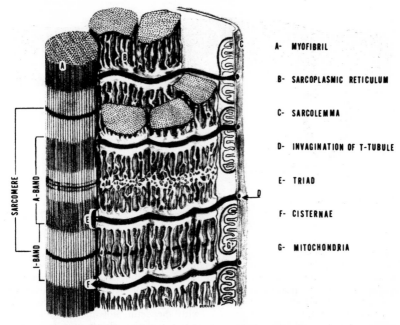

A- MYOFIBRIL

B- SARCOPLASMIC RETICULUM

C- SARCOLEMMA

D- INVAGINATION OF T-TUBULE

E- TRIAD

F- CISTERNAE

G- MITOCHONDRIA

Figure 2. Schematic representation of the intracellular organization of a mammalian muscle fiber. The distribution of the transverse tubular system (T-system) and the sarcoplasmic reticulum (SR) are illustrated in relation to each other and to their location within the sarcomere. (A modified drawing after L.D. Peachey. 1965. J. Cell Biol. 25:222.)

sarcomere (Figure 2). This membrane system has similar electrical properties to that of the sarcolemma; therefore, the depolarization impulse can be transmitted via this tubular network to the inner most depths of the fiber. The other tubular system, i.e., the sarcoplasmic reticulum (SR), is an internal system with a longitudinal orientation, which forms a fishnet-like mesh around each sarcomere (Figure 2). The SR is in juxtaposition to the T-tubular system, forming a triad arrangement. The SR contains a high concentration of calcium ions used for the initiation of muscle contraction. In brief, the events that lead to muscle contraction include the propagation of the electrical impulse, which was initially passed across the neuromuscular junction, along the sarcolemma and down the T-system to the level of the A-I junction of the sarcomere. This impulse influences the SR to release its calcium ions into the sarcoplasm. Calcium ions then bind to the troponin-tropomyosin complex associated with the actin filament. This regulatory protein complex then removes its inhibitory action, allowing interaction of the myosin cross-bridge with the actin filament. Thus

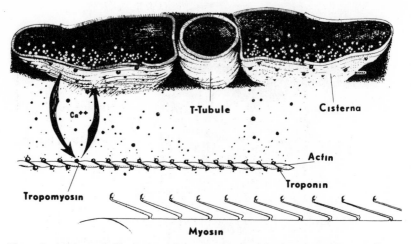

Figure 3. A schematic illustration of the process of excitation-contraction coupling. As an electrical impulse is propagated along the transverse tubule the sarcoplasmic reticulum (SR) releases its concentrated stores of calcium ions. These calcium ions diffuse into the sarcoplasm and bind with the troponin of the troponin–tropomyosin complex, thus releasing the pre-existing inhibition from the actin filament. The myosin cross-bridges can then interact with the actin protein. The process of relaxation occurs with the active re-sequestering of the calcium ions by the SR, allowing the troponin-tropomyosin complex to re-establish the inhibition of the actin filament.

muscle contraction is is initiated by activating the contractile proteins and ATP hydrolysis. Muscle relaxation occurs following the passage of the electrical impulse, at which time calcium ions are removed from the sarcoplasm by being actively re-sequestered by the SR. These events are illustrated in Figure 3.

Ultrastructural Characteristics

Ultrastructural studies have found differences in the neuromuscular junction of slow- and fast-twitch muscle fibers in lower mammals (23). Muscle fibers with fast-twitch characteristics have been observed to be innervated by nerves with a large, flat axonal ending containing a high concentration of acetylcholine vesicles (Figure 4). In contrast, slow-twitch fibers have a small, more rounded axonal ending with fewer vesicles. The endplate regions of fast-twitch fibers have deeper, more abundant and regular invaginations than slow-twitch fibers. The SR of fast-twitch fibers forms a more extensive network with a greater development of the terminal cisternae than found in slow-twitch fibers (23, 60). In addition to the SR of the slow-twitch fibers having a lesser development, their terminal

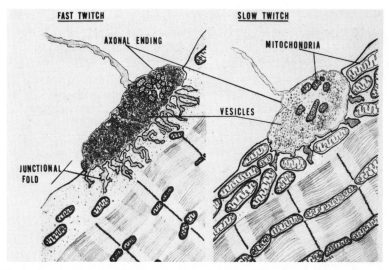

Figure 4. A comparative illustration of the neuromuscular junctions of slow- and fast-twitch muscle fibers. The neuromuscular junction of a fast-twitch muscle fiber can be noted to have a larger axonal ending, containing more vesicles, and a greater number of endplate junctional folds. Differences in fast- and slow-twitch muscle fibers are described in the text. (Illustrated after H.A. Padykula and G.F. Gauthier. 1970. J. Cell Biol. 46:27.)

cisternae have often been observed to flank the T-system only on one side, resulting in a dyad instead of the familiar triad arrangement (60). The slow-twitch fibers contain mitochondria that are larger and have a greater concentration of cristae than those in fast-twitch fibers. In this fiber type the mitochondria are often found in a continuous chain between the myofibrils and are particularly plentiful beneath the sarcolemma. In contrast, fast-twitch fibers have fewer and smaller mitochondria, often found in pairs at the level of the Z-line.

Studies using muscles from man have found ultrastructural differences in the fiber types similar to those observed in other species, namely in the number, form, and distribution of mitochondria, and in the neuromuscular junction (Table 1) (47, 49, 61). A prominent feature of the slow-twitch fiber are the long chains of large diameter mitochondria in the intermyofibrillar space, as well as numerous subsarcolemmal aggregates of mitochondria (as shown in Figure 4). The fast-twitch fibers have fewer and smaller mitochondria. They are often found paired at the Z-line. In these fibers, subsarcolemmal accumulations of mitochondria are essentially absent. The structural difference in the neuromuscular junctions is another

Table 1. Characteristics of human muscle fiber types[a]

Muscle fiber characteristics	Muscle fiber type	
	Slow-twitch	Fast-twitch
Morphological		
Mitochondria	large; many	small; few
Neuromuscular junction	small; simple	large; complex
Sarcoplasmic reticulum	similar	similar
Metabolic[b]		
Glycogenesis	↑	↓
Glycogenolysis	↓	↑
Glycolysis	↓	↑
Fatty acid utilization	↑	↓
Krebs cycle and electron transport system	↑	↓
Ketone body oxidation	↑	↓
Protein metabolism	↑	↓
Blood supply	↑	↓
Myoglobin content	↑	↓
Contractile		
Contraction speed	↓	↑
Relaxation time	↑	↓
Force-velocity relation	slow/relative load	fast/relative load
Length-tension relation	similar	similar

[a]Findings not available from studies using human subjects have been extrapolated from findings using other mammals.

[b]Enzyme activities of the respective metabolic pathways as estimated by histochemical or biochemical analysis have been used as indicators of the capacity of the metabolic characteristics. Arrows indicate higher or lower comparative values.

distinguishing characteristic of the different fiber types. The neuromuscular junction of the fast-twitch fiber is the most complex, having a large, flat axonal ending and long, closely packed junctional folds, whereas the myoneural junction of the slow-twitch fiber is smaller with shorter and fewer junctional invaginations. In contrast to the striking differences observed in other animals, findings of human studies indicate only slight differences in the abundance of SR for the different fiber types.

Histochemical and Biochemical Characteristics

The histochemical stain directed at myofibrillar ATPases has been used as an indicator of the contractile properties of muscle fibers. This histochemical technique presents two distinct staining intensities (at pH 9.4) indicating the existence of two types of muscle cells. One type contains myofibrillar ATPases with a slow catalytic rate, while the second type has fast myofibrillar ATPases (Figure 5) (*19, 26*). Biochemical determinations carried out on animal muscles composed of mostly homogenous fibers have found fast-twitch fibers to contain a myosin ATPase enzyme with a catalytic rate 3—4 times greater than that of slow-twitch muscle fibers (*6, 52*). This difference in catalytic rate has a high correlation with the difference in contractile speeds (*14*). Differences in troponin activity may also contribute to the differences in contraction times (*22*).

The two human muscle fiber types identified by the histochemical stain for myofibrillar ATPases also have distinct metabolic characteristics (Table 1) (*26*). The main function of the metabolic machinery in normal active muscle cells is to supply energy, in the form of ATP, to the contractile apparatus. Muscle fibers having a relatively greater quantity of mitochondria contain correspondingly greater amounts of Krebs cycle and electron transport system enzymes. In the presence of oxygen these fibers have a greater potential to produce ATP and are referred to as oxidative or aerobic fibers. Muscle fibers having a relatively high oxidative capacity appear red in color, which is indicative of a high content of mitochondria, myoglobin, and blood supply. Human muscle fibers with low myofibrillar ATPase activity appear to possess a high oxidative capacity, as indicated by the histochemical stain for DPNH-diaphorase (Figure 5). Fibers with a high aerobic capacity, as indicated by animal studies, have a greater ability for fatty acid and ketone body utilization than do less oxidative fibers (*37, 50*). In contrast, fibers with a high myofibrillar ATPase activity have a lesser oxidative potential, but possess a greater glycolytic or anaerobic capacity to produce ATP than the slow-twitch fibers. Hence, when these fibers are active they rely heavily on carbohydrates in the form of glycogen as a substrate. These two fiber types are similar in cross-sectional area and glycogen content (*26*).

A third muscle fiber type has been identified in various other species (*48, 52*). This fiber type has a high myofibrillar ATPase activity, high glycolytic activity, and high oxidative capacity. This type of fiber does not exist in human skeletal muscle.

The nuclear bag and nuclear chain fibers from humans have recently been described (*62*). The histochemical characteristics of these two intrafusal fibers are most similar to the slow-twitch oxidative extrafusal fiber. However, they differ from the slow-twitch fibers by having a higher oxidative capacity and from the nuclear chain fibers by having a high myofibrillar ATPase activity.

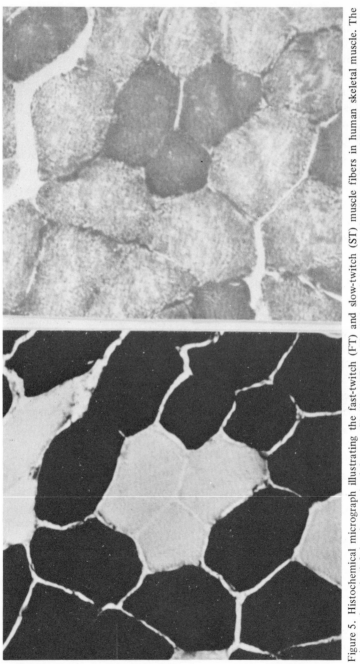

Figure 5. Histochemical micrograph illustrating the fast-twitch (FT) and slow-twitch (ST) muscle fibers in human skeletal muscle. The micrograph on the left has been stained for myofibrillar ATPase. The light and dark stained cells are ST and FT fibers, respectively. The micrograph at the right is from a serial section of the same muscle and has been stained for DPNH-diaphorase, which indicates the aerobic potential of the fibers. These micrographs illustrate that in human skeletal muscle ST fibers have a relatively high aerobic capacity, while FT fibers have a low capacity. (Micrographs by courtesy of Dr. Philip D. Gollnick.)

Contractile Characteristics of Different Fiber Types

The differences in the morphological and chemical characteristics of the muscle fiber types are reflected in their contractile expressions. The contractile characteristics of muscle are determined mainly by the following three factors: 1) duration of the active state, 2) force-velocity relation, and 3) length-tension relation.

The time course of the active state in fast-twitch muscles is markedly different from that of slow-twitch muscles (*14, 68*). In animals the contraction time (i.e., the time required to reach peak tension) has been determined to be 2—4 times quicker in fast than in slow muscles (Figure 6). Not until recently was it technically possible to directly determine the speed of contraction of the different fiber types in human muscles. The development of an indwelling needle transducer not only has allowed the direct determination of contraction times but also, in combination with histochemical analyses, has made possible the correlation of contractile properties with chemical characteristics. These findings suggest that fibers with slow-twitch times are rich in mitochondria and, conversely, that fast-twitch fibers have few mitochondria (*9, 10, 11*).

There are also differences in the time course of the relaxation period (i.e., the time required for the decay of the active state) of fast and slow muscles (Figure 6) (*14*). It been generally accepted that the active state of a muscle occurs when calcium ions are released from the SR into the

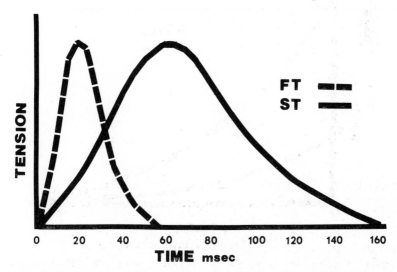

Figure 6. Contraction-relaxation curves for fast- (FT) and slow-twitch (ST) mammalian skeletal muscles.

sarcoplasm and bind with the troponin-tropomyosin complex, thereby removing the pre-existing inhibition imposed on the actin filament (Figure 3). The relaxation period has been shown to occur with the active re-sequestering of calcium ions by the SR, which allows the inhibition of the actin filament to be re-established. This has been supported by findings from animal studies indicating that the SR from fast muscle actively uptakes calcium ions several time faster than does that from slow muscle. Thus, the time differences for the events in the contraction-relaxation cycle of slow and fast muscles center on the differences in the catalytic rates of myofibrillar ATPases and on the exchange of calcium ions between troponin and the SR.

Differences in the force-velocity curves of fast- and slow-twitch muscles have been observed by using animal muscles that predominately consist of a single fiber type. The general qualitative character of the force-velocity relationship is similar for both fiber types (i.e., an increase in load results in a hyperbolic decrease in velocity). However, the curves are quantitatively different, with the rate of a shortening contraction being greater for fast-twitch muscles than that for slow-twitch muscles with the same relative load (Figure 7). The differences in the force-velocity proper-

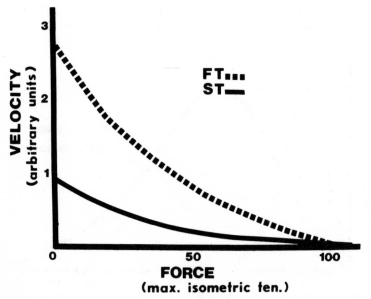

Figure 7. Force-velocity curves for fast- (FT) and slow-twitch (ST) mammalian skeletal muscles.

ties are related to the differences in the time course of the active state and to the catalytic rates of myofibrillar ATPases.

The length-tension relationships of slow and fast muscles are similar when the amount of force developed is expressed per unit of cross-sectional area (*14, 68*).

Physiological Roles of Slow and Fast Muscles

It is now known that muscle fibers within the same motor unit have similar histochemical profiles. Recently, direct evidence has been presented that associates the contractile properties with the histochemical characteristics of the different types of motor units (*12*). Motor units consisting of fibers with high myofibrillar ATPase activity and low oxidative capacity were found to have relatively fast contraction speeds and were quick to fatigue. Motor units of this type also have been found to have the greatest number of muscle fibers and the largest axonal diameters (Figure 8) (*34*). In contrast, motor units with fibers having low myofibrillar ATPase activity and high oxidative capacity are resistant to fatigue, slow contracting, and contain fewer muscle fibers. Furthermore, the slow-twitch motor units with small motoneurons are more susceptible to discharge and have a slower rate of impulse conduction than the larger

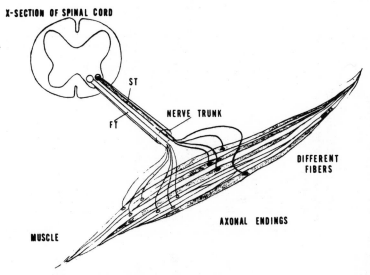

Figure 8. A schematic illustration of the fast- and slow-twitch motor units. The fast-twitch motor units are shown to have a larger axonal diameter and a greater innervation ratio than the slow-twitch units.

Table 2. Muscle fiber type classification systems

Fiber type terminology			Characteristic used for classification[a]	Species
white (fast-twitch white)	medium	red	ultrastructure	vertebrates (23)
A	B	C	metabolic	rat (62)
I	III	II	metabolic	rat and cat (53)
FTW (fast-twitch white)	STI (slow-twitch intermediate)	FTR (fast-twitch red)	contractile and metabolic	guinea pig (44)
LF (low-oxidative fast)	HS (high oxidative slow)	HF (high-oxidative fast)	contractile and metabolic	guinea pig (44)
FF (fast contracting-fast fatiguing)	S (slow contracting)	FR (fast contracting-fatigue resistant)	contractile, metabolic, and contractile times	cat (12)
α	β	αβ	contractile	rat (32)
FG (fast-twitch-glycolytic)	SO (slow-twitch-oxidative)	FOG (fast-twitch-oxidative-glycolytic)	contractile and metabolic	guinea pig and rabbit (52)
white	medium	red	metabolic	man, mouse, other vertebrates (48)
IIB	I	IIA	contractile	man, rat, rabbit (8)
α-white	β-red	α-red	contractile	man (2)
FT (fast-twitch)	ST (slow-twitch)	FT (fast-twitch)	contractile	man (26)
II	I (slow-twitch)		contractile	man (15, 20)
white	red		contractile	man (19)

[a]Characteristics used for establishing the classification systems are listed mainly as metabolic and contractile. For further details refer to the original article.

fast-twitch motor units. This ease of motor unit recruitment may further be related to the degree of utilization and possibly to the differentiation of contractile and metabolic characteristics. Anti-gravity muscles, e.g., soleus muscle, consist mainly of slow-twitch motor units and are considered to function tonically, e.g., during postural maintenance. Since slow-twitch muscle has been reported to be more efficient than fast-twitch muscle in maintaining isometric tension, this, combined with its high aerobic capacity, would best suit it for maintaining a static postural position (3). Muscles consisting mainly of fast motor units have been suggested to be more efficient during isotonic work and are believed to become active during voluntary phasic movements.

A preferential recruitment of motor units has been shown to occur in man during prolonged, moderately intense exercise (27). The histochemical determination of glycogen depletion has indicated that slow-twitch motor units are recruited at the commencement of prolonged, moderately intense exercise while fast-twitch fibers are recruited progressively over time. During high intensity exercise (150% of aerobic capacity) and voluntary isometric contraction (20% of maximal voluntary contraction and higher) the fast-twitch, along with the slow-twitch, units have been shown to be recruited immediately upon, or soon after, the commencement of exercise (27, 29).

Classification of Muscle Fiber Types

Numerous classification systems for muscle fiber types have been proposed, based on different contractile and metabolic muscle characteristics. An attempt has been made to compile a listing of the most widely used classification systems for the reader who is interested but unfamiliar with them (Table 2).

In general, two factors have been considered when establishing a classification system: 1) contractile properties and/or 2) metabolic characteristics. The contractile properties of muscle fibers are most often determined by histochemical staining techniques directed at myofibrillar ATPases, but bioassays of myosin ATPase and contractile times of homogenous whole muscles are also used. The metabolic characteristics have been determined using similar techniques directed at the levels of the oxidative and glycolytic capacities, which generally have an inverse relationship to each other in man. The separate application of these two factors, along with technique differences and interspecies variation, account in part for these numerous systems. The characteristic used as a basis for the classification of fibers is of utmost importance in the study of conditions of hypo- and hyper-function as well as in experiments involving pathological muscle.

The muscle cell has been shown to have considerable plasticity; therefore, for consistency, the most stable characteristic must be used in classification of fibers. In fact, the term "fiber type" has been objected to because it conveys an idea of stability to the characteristics of the muscle cell (33). It has been recommended that myofibrillar ATPases be used as a relatively stable characteristic that would reduce the variability in histochemical classification (20). Furthermore, they give a clear and constant separation of muscle fiber types into two distinct fiber populations and appear to be least changed in pathologic fibers. The less stable metabolic characteristics should serve in a supporting role as a descriptive adjective to the more stable contractile term. The metabolic term should indicate the relative oxidative and glycolytic potential of the cell.

PLASTICITY OF MUSCLE FIBER CHARACTERISTICS

In order to more fully understand the cellular processes of neuromuscular rehabilitation and exercise training, we must not only understand the character of the muscle fibers, but also be aware of conditions that can alter or maintain the characteristics of the muscle cell.

There is a continuing attempt to achieve a greater understanding of the factors that influence the differentiation of the contractile and metabolic properties of muscle fibers and, furthermore, to determine the extent to which these differentiated characteristics can be altered. There are two major mechanistic hypothesis: 1) Specific trophic substances may be produced by the motor neuron and passed on to the muscle cell. These postulated substances may then dictate the character of the muscle fiber by influencing gene expression. 2) A second hypothesis states that motor impulse traffic imposed on the muscle cell may require the development of specific fiber characteristics. An alternative to this hypothesis has stated that impulse traffic may first induce the production of a specific trophic substance by the motor neuron that is then transported to the muscle cell to induce specific differentiated characteristics as mentioned in the first hypothesis.

Cross-innervation

Cross-innervation experiments (i.e., cross-anastomosis of nerves from slow and fast muscles) dramatically demonstrate the importance of the nerve-muscle relationship (Figure 9). This experimental condition results in the complete reversal of the muscle's character (30, 32, 57, 58). Cross-innervated muscles originally having fast-twitch properties and low oxidative capacity take on slow-twitch characteristics and an increased oxidative capacity, while the inverse occurs for slow-twitch muscles innervated with nerves from fast muscles. The changes in the metabolic apparatus are accompanied by corresponding changes in the density of the capillaries surrounding the fibers. Besides demonstrating the plasticity of the capillary system in adapting to changing metabolic needs, this suggests the type of innervation can indirectly influence extracellular characteristics.

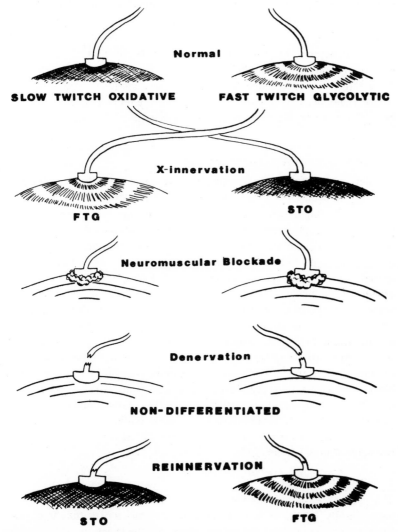

Figure 9. This is an illustration of selected experimental conditions used to alter the nerve-muscle relationship. See text for details.

Denervation

The importance of innervation to the muscle fiber has been further demonstrated by denervation experiments (Figure 9). When muscles are denervated, slow-twitch muscles increase slightly in speed of contraction, whereas fast-twitch muscles have a decrease in contractile speed (*31, 55*). The enzymes of energy metabolism in these muscles progressively decrease until the muscles become metabolically non-differentiated. Fibers with a high anaerobic potential have a more rapid reduction in glycolytic enzymes, while fibers high in oxidative capacity have the most rapid loss of oxidative enzymes. Localization of acetylcholine sensitivity to the motor endplate region is known to be maintained by the neural trophic influence. Denervation results in the development of extrajunctional hypersensitivity to acetylcholine. It is interesting to note that the time of development has been shown to be directly related to the length of the remaining nerve stump (*42*).

Neuromuscular and Axoplasmic Blockade

Further support for a trophic substance has come from the experimental use of a xylocaine nerve cuff, which produces a nerve impulse blockade without affecting axoplasmic flow. Findings obtained using this technique suggest that the prolonged absence of nerve impulses does not produce the development of membrane hypersensitivity to acetylcholine (*53*). Furthermore, muscle membrane hypersensitivity to acetylcholine has been reported following the application of drugs that block axoplasmic flow (*1*). These studies indicate that the trophic neural influence is independent of nerve impulses but dependent on axoplasmic substances. Although these findings have found impulse blockage to cause hypersensitivity and direct chronic stimulation of denervated fast or slow muscles to present denervation hypersensitivity (*41*), the establishment of a neuromuscular blockage by the administering of Clostridium botulinum toxin, a substance that blocks the release of acetylcholine while having no direct affect on the muscle, produces metabolic changes identical to those following denervation (Figure 9). It has been inferred from these findings that acetylcholine is the trophic "mysterine" that induces the differences in the metabolic character of muscle fibers (*55*).

Re-innervation

The re-innervation of denervated slow and fast muscles by their original nerve results in the return of the characteristic contractile times and force-velocity properties, and the metabolic redifferentiation of the muscle fibers (Figure 9) (*13, 55*). Although there is a re-establishment of the same proportion of fiber types in re-innervated muscles, small groups of homogeneous fibers exist, whereas in the normal muscles they are dispersed in a mosaic pattern throughout the muscle (*18*).

Immobilization and Tenotomy

Immobilization of an animal's limb or joint by pinning or casting, in addition to causing muscle atrophy, reduces the motor impulse traffic and has been observed to increase the speed of contraction in slow muscles with little or no change in contraction speed of fast muscles (*21, 31*). Immobilization does not seem to affect the metabolic characteristics of muscles of sedentary laboratory animals (*43*). Tenotomy and spinal cord transection produce effects similar to those of immobilization.

Electrical Stimulation

Although electrical stimulation is not strongly advised for clinical use it has been found to conserve certain characteristics of muscles. Prolonged electrical stimulation of a tenotomized muscle at frequencies mimicking normal impulse patterns of slow-twitch muscles have been found to conserve the muscle's slow contractile properties (*30, 66*). Support for the motor impulse theory has come from experiments that have imposed different patterns of stimulation on fast and slow muscles (*16, 56, 67*). Electrical stimulation of normal fast and slow muscles have indicated a tendency for slow muscle to increase contraction speed when chronically stimulated with impulse patterns similar to fast muscles, while the opposite occurs in fast muscle stimulated with impulse patterns of slow muscle.

Submaximal Exercise Training

It is well established that the physiological stimulus of physical exercise can modify skeletal muscle character. Prolonged, moderately intense exercise training induces adaptations in the cellular metabolic apparatus (*17, 39, 46, 51*). Endurance training induces increases in the size and number of mitochondria, with commensurate increases in Krebs cycle and electron transport enzymes (*28, 35*). These compensatory adaptations can double the aerobic capacity of skeletal muscle. The transport of oxygen to the mitochondria is facilitated by increases in myoglobin concentration following such training (*35*). The ability of the muscle cell to utilize fatty acids increases in proportion to the aerobic capacity (*45*).

Compensatory adaptations have also been reported in the enzyme pathways involved in carbohydrate metabolism. Exercise resulting in the depletion of muscle glycogen is followed by an increased storage of glycogen in the muscle, a phenomena termed "glycogen supercompensation" (*36*). Increases in the activities of enzymes involved in this process probably account for this overcompensation (*51, 65*). In addition, prolonged, submaximal training has been reported to induce increases in the enzyme pathway of glycogen catabolism (*64*). Though findings related to the effects of endurance training on the glycogenolytic and glycolytic capacity of skeletal muscle are controversial (*25, 35, 64*), recent investigations using man have reported increases in two regulatory enzymes involved in carbohydrate metabolism (i.e., phosphorylase and phosphofructokinase), which suggests an increased potential of trained muscle to utilize glucose (*25, 64*).

Histochemical and biochemical findings show that the increased oxidative capacity induced by endurance training is not fiber type specific, since the same relative increase in oxidative capacity has been found to occur in the different fiber types (*5*). The contractile characteristics of muscle are not altered by endurance training, as indicated by no change in myosin ATPase activities, in capacity of isolated SR to bind calcium ions, or in contraction and relaxation times (*4, 7*).

In summary, hyperfunction imposed on skeletal muscle by prolonged, moderately intense training has been observed to induce metabolic changes in the muscle cell that are not fiber type selective, while the contractile properties seem to be unaltered by this type of training. Although the physiological significance of these adaptations is not fully understood, present hypotheses center on the conservation of glycogen stores. The elevated aerobic capacity of the muscle cell allows for a greater reliance on fat metabolism at submaximal work levels, thus prolonging the time for glycogen depletion, which has a high correlation with fatigue during moderately intense exercise.

Compensatory Muscle Growth

The plasticity of muscle fiber characteristics is also being studied by inducing compensatory muscular enlargement in animals by tenotomy or surgical removal of a synergistic muscle (*24, 33*). Following the surgical elimination of the gastrocnemius muscle, dramatic increases in the size of the plantaris and soleus muscles have been observed (*33, 59*). The mechanism for this compensatory growth involves hypertrophy of each of the different muscle fiber types and possibly a hyperplasia of muscle cells. This type of hyperfunction has been shown to produce a shifting of the fiber type spectrum towards the slow-twitch-oxidative fibers (unpublished findings). The metabolic potential of the enlarged muscle is similar to that of normal muscle (unpublished findings). The consequences of the acute phase of muscle hypertrophy on contractile properties have been reported as a depression of tension developed per unit mass and an increase in contraction time (*40*).

SUMMARY

The above investigations have vividly demonstrated the importance of the nerve-muscle relationship and of the degree of plasticity of muscle cell characteristics. The theory of neural trophic substance(s) has received support from the cross-innervation, denervation, neuromuscular blockade, and re-innervation experiments, while support for impulse activity as a determinate of muscle fiber character has come from investigations using immobilization, tenotomy, spinal cord transection, and electrical stimulation. Separately, neither of these current hypotheses can fully explain all the findings, but a combination of these hypotheses may prove beneficial, since it has been suggested that impulse activity can influence axoplasmic flow (*38*). Physiological peripheral stimuli (i.e., metabolic and power overload conditions) also are known to have the ability to selectively alter characteristics of the muscle cell.

Health professionals must continue to pursue a greater understanding of the cellular characteristics of human muscle fiber types and the factors involved in determining these characteristics, in order to better understand the etiology, pathogenesis, diagnosis, and rehabilitation of neuromuscular disorders. A greater insight into muscle cell plasticity is a must for the rehabilitative therapist and persons involved in physical training, since it is the plastic property of skeletal muscle that is relied upon for neuromuscular rehabilitation and exercise training.

ACKNOWLEDGMENT

Figures 1, 2, 3, 4, 8, and 9 were drawn by Ms. Lorraine Bernier Berry.

LITERATURE CITED

1. Albuquerque, E.X., J.E. Warnick, J.R. Tasse, and F.M. Sansone. 1972. Effects of vinblastine and colchicine on neural regulation of the fast and slow skeletal muscles of the rat. Exp. Neurol. 37:607–634.
2. Ashmore, C.R., and L. Doerr. 1971. Comparative aspects of muscle fiber types in different species. Exp. Neurol. 31:408–418.
3. Awan, M.Z., and G. Goldspink. 1970. Energy utilization by mammalian fast and slow muscle in doing external work. Biochim. Biophys. Acta 216:229–230.
4. Bagby, G.J., W.L. Sembrowich, and P.D. Gollnick. 1972. Myosin

ATPase and fiber composition from trained and untrained rat skeletal muscle. Am. J. Physiol. 223:1415–1417.

5. Baldwin, K.M., G.M. Klinkerfuss, R.L. Terjung, and P.A. Molé. 1972. Respiratory capacity of white, red, and intermediate muscle: adaptative response to exercise. Am. J. Physiol. 222:373–378.

6. Barnard, R.J., V.R. Edgerton, T. Furukawa, and J.B. Peter. 1971. Histochemical, biochemical, and contractile properties of red, white, and intermediate fibers. Am. J. Physiol. 220:410–414.

7. Barnard, R.J., V.R. Edgerton, and J.B. Peter. 1970. Effects of exercise on skeletal muscle I. Biochemical and histochemical properties. J. Appl. Physiol. 28:762–766.

8. Brooke, M.H., and K.K. Kaiser. 1970. Muscle fiber types: how many and what kind? Arch. Neurol. 23:369–379.

9. Buchthal, F., and H. Schmalbruch. 1969. Spectrum of contraction times of different fiber bundles in the brachial biceps and triceps muscles of man. Nature 222:89.

10. Buchthal, F., and H. Schmalbruch. 1970. Contraction times and fiber types in intact human muscle. Acta Physiol. Scand. 79:435–452.

11. Buchthal, F., H. Schmalbruch, and A. Kamieniecka. 1971. Contraction times and fiber types in patients with progressive muscular dystrophy. Neurology 21:131–139.

12. Burke, R.E., D.N. Levine, and F.E. Zajac, III. 1971. Mammalian motor units: physiological-histochemical correlation in three types in cat gastrocnemius. Science 174:709–712.

13. Close, R.I. 1969. Dynamic properties of fast and slow skeletal muscles of the rat after nerve cross-union. J. Physiol. 204:331–346.

14. Close, R.I. 1972. Dynamic properties of mammalian skeletal muscles. Physiol. Rev. 51:129–197.

15. Dubowitz, A., and A.G. Everson Pearse. 1960. A comparative histochemical study of oxidative enzyme and phosphorylase activity in skeletal muscle. Histochemie 2:105–117.

16. Eccles, J.C., R.M. Eccles, and W. Kozak. 1962. Further investigations on the influence of motoneurones on the speed of muscle contraction. J. Physiol. 163:324–339.

17. Edgerton, V.R., L. Gerchman, and R. Carrow. 1969. Histochemical changes in rat skeletal muscle after exercise. Exp. Neurol. 24:110–123.

18. Edstrom, L., and E. Kugelberg. 1969. Histochemical mapping of motor units in experimentally re-innervated skeletal muscle. Experientia 25:1044–1045.

19. Edstrom, L., and B. Nystrom. 1969. Histochemical types and sizes of fibres in normal human muscles. Acta Neurol. Scand. 45:257–269.

20. Engel, W.K. 1970. Selective and nonselective susceptibility of muscle fiber types. Arch. Neurol. 22:97–117.

21. Fischbach, G.D., and N. Robbins. 1969. Changes in contractile properties of disused soleus muscles. J. Physiol. 201:305–320.

22. Furukawa, T., and J.B. Peter. 1971. Troponin activity of different types of muscle fibers. Exp. Neurol. 31:214–222.

23. Gauthier, G.F. 1971. The structural and cytochemical heterogeneity

of mammalian skeletal muscle fibers. *In* R.J. Podolsky (ed.), Contractility of Muscle Cells and Related Processes. Prentice-Hall, New Jersey. pp. 131–150.

24. Goldberg, A.L. 1971. Biochemical events during hypertrophy of skeletal muscle. *In* N.R. Alpert (ed.), Cardiac Hypertrophy. Academic Press, New York. pp. 301–314.

25. Gollnick, P.D., R.B. Armstrong, B. Saltin, C.W. Saubert IV, W.L. Sembrowich, and R.E. Shephard. 1973. Effect of training on enzyme activity and fiber composition of human skeletal muscle. J. Appl. Physiol. 34:107–111.

26. Gollnick, P.D., R.B. Armstrong, C.W. Saubert IV, K. Piehl, and B. Saltin. 1972. Enzyme activity and fiber composition in skeletal muscle of untrained and trained men. J. Appl. Physiol. 33:312–319.

27. Gollnick, P.D., R.B. Armstrong, W.L. Sembrowich, R.E. Shephard, and B. Saltin. 1973. Glycogen depletion pattern in human skeletal muscle fibers after heavy exercise. J. Appl. Physiol. 34:615–618.

28. Gollnick, P.D., C.D. Ianuzzo, and D.W. King. 1971. Ultrastructural and enzyme changes in muscles with exercise. *In* B. Pernow and B. Saltin (eds.), Muscle Metabolism During Exercise. Plenum, New York. pp. 69–85.

29. Gollnick, P.D., J. Karlson, and B. Saltin. 1973. Glycogen depletion in human skeletal muscle fibers during isometric exercise. Physiologist 16:325.

30. Guth, L. 1968. "Trophic" influences of nerve on muscle. Physiol. Rev. 48:645–687.

31. Guth, L. 1970. "Trophic" effects of vertebrate neurons. *In* F.O. Schmitt, T. Melnechuk, G. Quarton, and G. Adelman (eds.), Neurosciences Research Symposium Summaries. M.I.T. Press, Cambridge, Mass. pp. 327–396.

32. Guth, L., F.J. Samaha, and R.W. Albers. 1970. The neural regulation of some phenotypic differences between the fiber types of mammalian skeletal muscle. Exp. Neurol. 26:126–135.

33. Guth, L., and H. Yellin. 1971. The dynamic nature of the so-called "fiber types" of mammalian skeletal muscle. Exp. Neurol. 31:277–300.

34. Henneman, E., and C.B. Olson. 1965. Relations between structure and function in the design of skeletal muscles. J. Neurophysiol. 28:581–598.

35. Holloszy, J.O., L.B. Oscai, P.A. Mole, and I.J. Don. 1971. Biochemical adaptations to endurance exercise in skeletal muscle. *In* B. Pernow and B. Saltin (eds.), Muscle Metabolism During Exercise. Plenum, New York. pp. 51–61.

36. Hultman, E., T. Bergstrom, and A.E. Roch-Norbund. 1971. Glycogen storage in human skeletal muscle. *In* B. Pernow and B. Saltin, (eds.), Muscle Metabolism During Exercise, Plenum, New York. pp. 273–288.

37. Kark, R.A.P., J.P. Blass, J. Avigan, and W.K. Engel. 1971. The oxidation of B-hydroxybutyric acid by small quantities of type-pure red and white skeletal muscle. J. Biol. Chem. 246:4560–4566.

38. Kerkut, G.A., A. Shapiro, and R.J. Walker. 1967. The transport of [14] C-labelled material from CNS to muscle along a nerve trunk. Comp. Biochem. Physiol. 23:729–748.
39. Kiessling, K.H., K. Piehl, and C.G. Lundquist. 1971. Effect of physical training on ultrastructural features in human skeletal muscle. *In* B. Pernow and B. Saltin (eds.), Muscle Metabolism During Exercise, Plenum, New York. pp. 97–102.
40. Lesch, M. 1971. Effects of acute hypertrophy on the contractile properties of skeletal muscle. *In* N.R. Alpert (ed.), Cardiac Hypertrophy, Academic Press, New York. pp. 147–155.
41. Lomo, T., and J. Rosenthal. 1972. Control of ACh sensitivity by muscle activity in the rat. J. Physiol. 221:493–513.
42. Luco, J.V., and C. Eyzaquirre. 1955. Fibrillation and hypersensitivity to ACh in denervated muscle: effect of length of degenerating nerve fibers. J. Neurophysiol. 18:65–73.
43. Mann, W.S., and B. Salafasky. 1970. Enzymic and physiological studies on normal and disused developing fast and slow cat muscles. J. Physiol. 208:33–47.
44. Maxwell, L.C., J.A. Faulkner, and D.A. Lieberman. 1973. Histochemical manifestations of age and endurance training in skeletal muscle fibers. Am. J. Physiol. 224:356–361.
45. Mole, P.A., K.M. Baldwin, R.L. Terjung, and J.O. Holloszy. 1973. Enzymatic pathways of pyruvate metabolism in skeletal muscle: adaptations to exercise. Am. J. Physiol. 224:50–54.
46. Morgan, T.E., L.A. Cobb, F.A. Short, R. Ross, and D.R. Gunn. 1971. Effects of long-term exercise on human muscle mitochondria. *In* B. Pernow and B. Saltin (eds.), Muscle Metabolism During Exercise. Plenum, New York. pp. 87–95.
47. Murata, F., and T. Ogata. 1969. The ultrastructure of neuromuscular junctions of human red, white and intermediate striated muscle fibers. Tohoku J. Exp. Med. 99:289–301.
48. Ogata, T., and M. Mori. 1964. Histochemical study of oxidative enzymes in vertebrate muscle. J. Histochem. Cytochem. 12:171–182.
49. Ogata, T., and F. Murata. 1969. Cytological features of three fiber types in human striated muscle. Tohoku J. Exp. Med. 99:225–245.
50. Pande, S.V., and M.S. Blanchaer. 1971. Carbohydrate and fat in energy metabolism of red and white muscle. Am. J. Physiol. 220:549–553.
51. Peter, J.B. 1971. Histochemical, biochemical, and physiological studies of skeletal muscle and its adaptation to exercise. *In* R.J. Podolsky (ed.), Contractility of Muscle Cells and Related Processes. Prentice-Hall, New Jersey. pp. 151–173.
52. Peter, J.B., R.J. Barnard, V.R. Edgerton, C.A. Gillespie, and K.E. Stempel. 1972. Metabolic profiles of three fiber types of skeletal muscle in guinea pigs and rabbits. Biochemistry 11:2627–2634.
53. Robert, E.D., and Y.T. Oester. 1970. Nerve impulses and trophic effect. Arch. Neurol. 22:27–63.

54. Romanul, F.C.A. 1964. Enzymes in muscle. I. Histochemical studies of enzymes in individual muscle fibers. Arch. Neurol. 11:355–369.
55. Romanul, F.C.A. 1971. Reversal of enzymatic profiles and capillary supply of muscles in fast and slow muscles after cross innervation. *In* B. Pernow and B. Saltin (eds.), Muscle Metabolism During Exercise. Plenum, New York. pp. 21–32.
56. Salmons, S., and G. Vrbova. 1969. The influence of activity on some contractile characteristics of mammalian fast and slow muscles. J. Physiol. 201:535–549.
57. Samaha, F.J., L. Guth, and R.W. Albers. 1970. The neural regulation of gene expression in the muscle cell. Exp. Neurol. 27:276–282.
58. Samaha, F.J., L. Guth, and R.W. Albers. 1970. Differences between slow and fast muscle myosin. J. Biol. Chem. 245:219–224.
59. Schiaffino, S., and S.P. Bormioli. 1973. Adaptive changes in developing rat skeletal muscle in response to functional overload. Exp. Neurol. 40:126–137.
60. Schiaffino, S., V. Hanzlikova, and S. Pierobon. 1970. Relations between structure and function in rat skeletal muscle fibers. J. Cell. Bio. 47:107–119.
61. Shafig, S.A., M. Gorycki, L. Goldstone, and A.T. Milhorat. 1966. Fine structure of fiber types in normal human muscle. Anat. Rec. 156:283–302.
62. Spiro, A.J., and R.L. Beibin. 1969. Human muscle spindle histochemistry. Arch. Neurol. 20:271–275.
63. Stein, J.M., and H.A. Padykula. 1962. Histochemical classification of individual skeletal muscle fibers of the rat. Am. J. Anat. 110:103–124.
64. Taylor, A.W., M.A. Booth, and S. Rao. 1972. Human skeletal muscle phosphorylase activities with exercise and training. Can. J. Physiol. Pharmacol. 50:1038–1042.
65. Taylor, A.W., R. Thayer, and S. Rao. 1971. Human skeletal muscle glycogen synthetase activities with exercise and training. Can. J. Physiol. Pharmacol. 50:411–415.
66. Vrbova, G. 1963. The effect of motoneurone activity on the speed of contraction of striated muscle. J. Physiol. 169:513–526.
67. Vrbova, G. 1966. Factors determining the speed of contraction of striated muscle. J. Physiol. 185:17.
68. Wells, J.B. 1965. Comparison of mechanical properties between slow and fast mammalian muscles. J. Physiol. 178:252–269.

ENERGY RELEASE IN THE EXTRAFUSAL MUSCLE FIBER

Robert B. Armstrong

SIGNIFICANCE OF ATP IN THE MUSCLE CELL

A number of vital biochemical processes in muscle cells require energy. These interactions are endergonic, which simply means that for the reaction to proceed, energy must be provided from another source. Muscle contraction is an obvious example of an endergonic biochemical interaction; movement of the thin filaments past the thick filaments during active muscle shortening requires energy.

Though energy exists in a variety of forms in nature, living cells depend upon the chemical energy contained in complex organic molecules. Some chemical energy is stored in all molecules, but most cellular processes obtain their energy from a specific high energy compound, adenosine triphosphate (ATP). The ATP molecule is composed of a nucleoside (ribose sugar and adenine base) and three phosphoric acid groups (Figure 1). The available chemical energy is stored in the ATP molecule so that hydrolysis, or splitting, of either of the terminal phosphates from the molecule releases energy that may be used to power endergonic cellular reactions. ATP is generally hydrolyzed to adenosine diphosphate (ADP) and inorganic phospate (P_i) in an exergonic (energy-releasing) reaction catalyzed by an adenosine triphosphatase (ATPase) enzyme. This reaction is summarized in the following equation:

$$ATP + H_2O \xrightarrow{ATPase} ADP + P_i + energy$$

Hydrolysis of the terminal phosphate group releases about 7.6 kcal of energy per mole of ATP under standardized laboratory conditions. How-

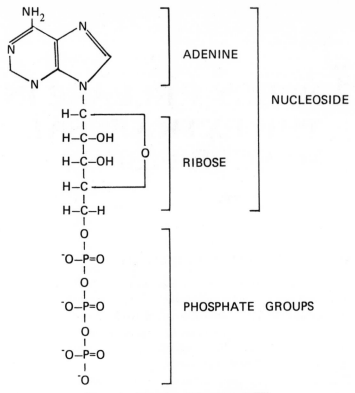

Figure 1. Adenosine triphosphate (ATP).

ever, under normal intracellular conditions in the muscle fiber, a free energy change of as much as 12 kcal per mole of ATP may occur.

In the muscle cell, ATP is required for a number of vital processes, e.g., synthesis of proteins, maintenance of the membrane potential, active transport of Ca^{2+} into the sarcoplasmic reticulum, and contraction. Although ATP is necessary for all of these functions, the following discussion will focus on the energy requirements for contraction.

ATP REQUIREMENTS IN MUSCLE CONTRACTION

The fundamental process of muscle contraction involves an interaction between actin and myosin protein molecules. During active contraction the association of these proteins is accompanied by hydrolysis of ATP to ADP and P_i. Removal of the terminal phosphate from ATP releases the stored chemical energy needed to power the contractile process. Though it is not the purpose of this article to discuss the mechanics or energetics of muscle contraction, the following outline is presented to summarize present understanding of ATP utilization in the contractile process. ATP function in contraction was described in a recent review (11).

In the resting muscle, ATP and magnesium ion (Mg^{2+}) are bound to the portion of myosin that forms the cross-bridge with actin during contraction. Most of the myosin · ATP · Mg^{2+} complex exists in an activated intermediate form that displays a great affinity for actin. The binding of the complex with actin is prevented by the inhibitory influence of troponin (through tropomyosin), a protein associated with the actin, or thin, filament. Calcium ions (Ca^{2+}) released by the sarcoplasmic reticulum following neural activation of the fiber bind to troponin, causing it to relinquish its inhibitory effect, and the myosin · ATP · Mg^{2+} complex interacts with actin. Upon binding with actin, the ATPase located on the myosin cross-bridge catalyzes the hydrolysis of ATP to ADP and P_i. This reaction releases the energy necessary for the cross-bridge to "pull" the thin filament, so that the Z line is drawn toward the center of the sarcomere. When the movement of the cross-bridge is completed, it is necessary for the bond between the filaments to be broken so that the cross-bridge may return to its normal position, reattach, and again exert tension on the actin. This "rowing" effect is possible because after the cross-bridge has completed its movement, a new ATP molecule binds to the actin · myosin · ADP complex releasing the ADP molecule, and causing the myosin cross-bridge to detach from the actin filament. Thus, the cycle is completed and the myosin · ATP · Mg^{2+} complex is again ready to interact with actin. As long as the Ca^{2+} concentration in the myofibril is adequate to prevent inhibition by troponin, the cycle is repeated and the thin filament is successively drawn toward the sarcomere's center.

In the absence of ATP, the actin · myosin · ADP complex cannot be broken, and the muscle is unable to relax. This explains the static contracture, referred to as rigor, that is observed in dying muscle tissue. Thus, ATP serves two distinct roles in the contraction-relaxation cycle in muscle: 1) to power the shortening process, and 2) to break the actin-myosin bond, allowing relaxation of the cross-bridge. An adequate supply of the high energy compound is therefore essential for normal contractile function.

ATP PRODUCTION

Immediate Sources of ATP

Muscle fibers do not obtain ATP from an extracellular source. Most essential substances are transported to the muscle by the circulating blood (e.g., amino acids, fatty acids, glucose, and oxygen), but the level of free ATP in blood is negligible and the compound does not readily diffuse through the cell membrane. Also, the amount of ATP stored in the cell is slight. In human vastus lateralis muscle at rest, ATP concentration is about 25 μmol per gram dry weight of muscle (6). Care must be observed in relating data from experimental animal preparations to the in vivo condition in man, but comparisons may be made to approximate the amount of contractile activity that can be supported by the stored ATP in the cell. Single twitches of frog sartorius muscle result in hydrolysis of about 0.3 μmol of ATP per gram of muscle (9). Assuming a similar rate of ATP breakdown in human muscle, the concentration found in vastus lateralis muscle should be sufficient to support approximately 85 twitches. It may be appreciated that during vigorous muscular exercise this level of ATP is inadequate for more than a few brief bursts of activity. There also is evidence that ATP is compartmentalized within the cell, which suggests that only a fraction of the total content is available for contractile activity (5). The fiber must therefore possess the inherent potential to replace the ATP as it is utilized.

One mechanism by which ATP is regenerated during muscular activity is through a reaction catalyzed by the enzyme creatine kinase. In this process the high energy phosphate of creatine phosphate (CP) is transferred to the ADP formed from ATP hydrolysis during contraction. This reaction may be summarized as follows:

$$CP + ADP \underset{\text{ATP-creatine transphosphorylase}}{\overset{\text{creatine kinase}}{\rightleftharpoons}} C + ATP$$

This transfer is immediate, and is the most important means of resynthesizing ATP during bursts of muscular activity. However, the concentration of CP in the cell is also quite low. In human vastus lateralis muscle the CP concentration is about 70 μmol per gram dry weight of muscle (6). The combined energy stored in ATP and CP in muscle fibers is therefore only adequate for brief periods of activity, and not for muscular activity of longer duration. CP is resynthesized from C and ATP in a reaction catalyzed by ATP-creatine transphosphorylase when sufficient ATP is available in the cell.

Another enzyme present in muscle cells, myokinase, catalyzes the production of ATP from two molecules of ADP as follows:

$$2 \text{ ADP} \xrightarrow{\text{myokinase}} \text{AMP} + \text{ATP}$$

Though this reaction is probably of little importance under normal conditions, it may become significant during intense muscular activity. The AMP produced in this process may also play an important role in stimulating other enzymes involved in energy production (e.g., phosphofructokinase).

The creatine kinase and myokinase reactions provide short-term high energy phosphate reserves for ATP resynthesis, but the respective reactants must eventually be resynthesized from ATP. Phosphorylation of creatine occurs at the expense of ATP, and reconversion of AMP to ADP utilizes the terminal phosphate of ATP. Therefore, ATP synthesis ultimately depends on energy derived from the breakdown of nutritive molecules in several complex enzymatic pathways in the cell. As indicated above, muscle cannot receive ATP from an outside source, so individual fibers must possess these metabolic systems.

Oxidative Phosphorylation

More than 90% of the ATP production in the muscle cell occurs in the mitochondria (Figure 2). Though differences in the distribution of mito-

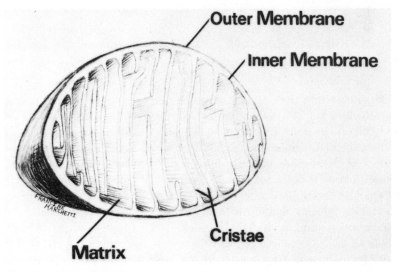

Figure 2. Schematic illustration of a mitochondrion.

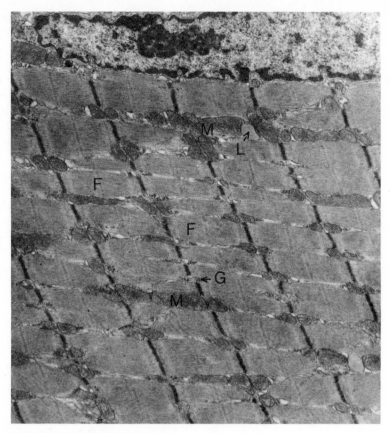

Figure 3a.

chondria within the cell exist among different types of skeletal muscle fibers, they are always found in the sarcoplasm in close proximity to the myofibrils where ATP is needed to power contraction (Figure 3). A mitochondrion consists of two membranes and a central fluid matrix. The inner membrane has numerous infoldings, or cristae. It is on these structures that most of the enzymes involved in ATP production are located. In particular, there are numerous series of ordered molecules capable of receiving reducing equivalents (hydrogen and electrons) from other metabolic sources and sequentially transferring them from molecule to molecule to a final combination with oxygen to form water (Figure 4). The passage of reducing equivalents among these molecules (coenzymes and cytochromes) is accomplished by reduction (electron gain) and reoxida-

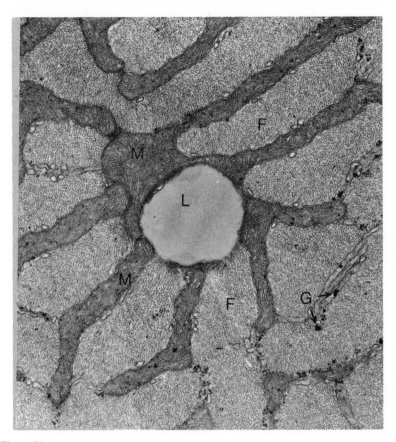

Figure 3*b*.

Figure 3. Electron micrographs illustrating the relationship between mitochondria (M) and the contractile elements of the muscle fiber, the myofibrils (F). Note the glycogen particles (G) and lipid droplets (L) interspersed among the myofibrils. Figure 3*a* is a longitudinal section through a fiber from rat plantaris muscle. ×14,000. (Courtesy of T. Chao and J. Albright). Figure 3*b* is a transverse section of a fiber from soleus muscle of hamster. ×28,000. (Courtesy of S. Anapolle and J. Albright). Note the way the mitcochondria almost completely surround some myofibrils in the cross-section.

tion (electron loss) of each successive member of the chain. These chemical changes are accompanied by the release of relatively large amounts of energy. The mitochondrion is able to utilize the energy released in the electron transport chain to bind P_i to ADP. Under normal conditions, two or three molecules of ATP are produced for every pair of electrons (or hydrogen atoms) that pass down the respiratory chain, depending on

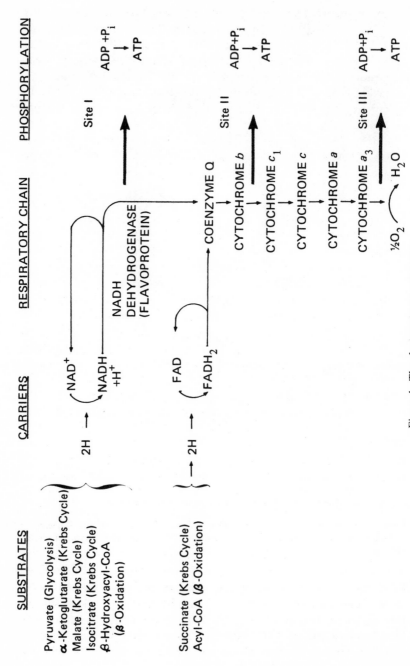

Figure 4. The electron transport system.

where the reducing equivalents enter the chain. A hydrogen pair transferred to the electron transport system by flavin adenine dinucleotide (FAD) produces only two molecules of ATP because it bypasses the first site of phosphorylation (Site I), whereas reducing equivalents entering through nicatinomide adenine dinucleotide (NAD^+) pass all three sites.

Production of ATP with energy derived from oxidation in the electron transport system is referred to as oxidative phosphorylation. For each pair of hydrogens that combines with an atom of oxygen to form H_2O at the end of the chain there are normally either two or three ATP molecules formed, depending on whether or not the hydrogens pass Site I. Thus, the ratio of ATP formed to oxygen consumed, the P:O ratio, is between 2 and 3 in the muscle cell (normally about 2.7).

Respiratory rate and the rate at which ATP is formed by the electron transport chain are normally controlled by the concentration of ADP in the muscle cell. The total amount of nucleotide in the cell remains fairly constant, i.e., the sum of ATP, ADP, and AMP does not change. However, the relative amounts of these nucleotides change depending upon the energetic condition of the muscle fiber. During rest the nucleotide primarily exists as ATP, with a reciprocally low level of ADP. However, muscular activity involves an increased hydrolysis of ATP so that the ADP content in the fiber rises. The availability of ADP in turn allows the mitochondrion to respire at an elevated rate to replenish ATP and the O_2 consumption rises in the cell. Normally, phosphorylation is tightly coupled to oxidation so that respiration in the mitochondrion cannot occur without phosphorylation of ADP.

Though the transfer of reducing equivalents through the electron transport system affects the major portion of ATP synthesis in the muscle fiber, ATP is also formed in other metabolic enzyme pathways. Moreover, it is necessary to consider the sources of the reducing equivalents utilized in the respiratory chain.

Production of Reducing Equivalents

Like most animal cells, muscle fibers do not possess the capacity to produce the basic nutritional energy-containing molecules that are necessary for ATP production. These organic dietary substances are ultimately derived from glucose produced by plant photosynthetic processes. Thus, the original source of all complex nutrients (proteins, fats, and carbohydrates) used in the muscle cell for energy production is plant glucose. Human diet consists primarily of the complex foodstuffs, and the muscle fiber possesses the metabolic capacity to utilize elements of all three types for ATP production. In a healthy individual, the nutritional substrate metabolized by the muscle cell at any particular time is primarily dictated by the degree of contractile activity of the fiber or the muscle as a whole. In the resting condition, or during periods of light to moderate activity, blood supply to the muscle fiber is adequate to supply oxygen for mitochondrial respiration and to provide sufficient plasma-transported substrates, particularly free fatty acids (FFA) and glucose. Under these conditions, the primary energy substrate in muscle is FFA.

FFA Metabolism

There are several long chain fatty acids that are metabolized by the muscle cell. Oleic acid $(CH_3(CH_2)_7CH = CH(CH_2)_7COO^-)$ is the most concentrated of the FFA in the blood and therefore experiences the greatest uptake by muscle fibers (4). In fact, uptake of all FFA by muscle cells is directly proportional to their concentrations in the blood, so that availability of this particular substrate to the fiber apparently dictates its extraction by the muscle.

β-oxidation   After entering the muscle cell, FFA are activated in the sarcoplasm with energy obtained from breakdown of ATP to AMP and PP_i in a reaction catalyzed by thiokinase (Figure 5). In this process the fatty acid is complexed with Coenzyme A. The activated fatty acid is then transported into the mitochondrion where its subsequent catabolism results in the sequential removal of 2-carbon fragments from the fatty acid as acetyl-CoA. This cyclic metabolic process is referred to as β-oxidation. In the process of removal of the acetyl fragments, two of the reactions involve dehydrogenations with the production of reducing equivalents. In the first, a flavoprotein serves as the hydrogen carrier, and in the second, NAD^+ is the cofactor. These reducing equivalents are then transferred to the respiratory chain for ATP production by oxidative phosphorylation (Figure 4). The acetyl-CoA produced in β-oxidation may then enter a second enzyme pathway (Krebs cycle) in which the 2-carbon fragment is completely oxidized to CO_2 and reducing equivalents. Several intermediate conversions are also required in the production of the acetyl-CoA from the fragment that contains the single double bond during the β-oxidation of oleic acid.

Krebs Cycle   In the first reaction of the Krebs cycle (Figure 6), acetyl-CoA condenses with oxalacetate to form citrate. Citrate is then oxidized in a series of reactions with the production of reducing equivalents, CO_2, and oxalacetate. Oxidation of one molecule of acetyl-CoA in the Krebs cycle results in 2 molecules of CO_2 so that one complete cycle regenerates the oxalacetate, which, along with acetyl-CoA, was one of the original reactants. There is also a net of 3 molecules of H_2O added during

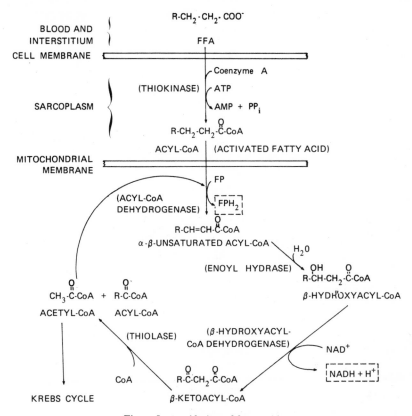

Figure 5. β-oxidation of fatty acids.

the cycle. In one specific step in the cycle, P_i is added to ADP to form ATP (succinate thiokinase reaction). Because this process does not occur in the respiratory chain, it is referred to as "phosphorylation at the substrate level." The net reaction of the Krebs cycle is represented in the following equation:

$$\text{acetyl-CoA} + 3NAD^+ + FAD + 3H_2O + ADP + P_i \rightarrow CoA + 2CO_2 + 3NADH + 3H^+ + FADH_2 + ATP$$

Catabolism of the fatty acid produces 2 pairs of reducing equivalents for every cycling of the molecule through β-oxidation to acetyl-CoA, and the oxidation of each resulting acetyl-CoA molecule in the Krebs cycle generates 4 pairs of hydrogens and one molecule of ATP. The fatty acids are composed of long carbon chains, so that these processes are repeated many times during oxidation of one FFA molecule. Oxidation of one

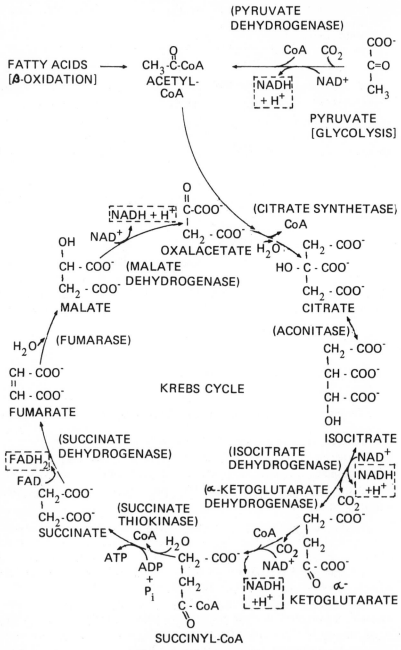

Figure 6. The Krebs cycle.

activated oleic acid molecule in β-oxidation and the Krebs cycle is summarized in the following equation:

$$\text{Oleic acid} + 17FAD + 35NAD^+ + 9ADP + 9P_i \rightarrow 18CO_2 + AMP + PP_i + 17FADH_2 + 35NADH + 35H^+ + 7ATP$$

Each of the molecules of NADH formed during β-oxidation and oxidation in the Krebs cycle will result in 3 molecules of ATP produced in the respiratory chain, and each molecule of $FADH_2$ will allow 2 ATP to be formed. Therefore, $(35 \times 3\ ATP) + (17 \times 2\ ATP) + (9\ ATP$ formed at the substrate level) = 148 ATP produced from one molecule of activated oleate.

Initial activation of the fatty acid is accompanied by hydrolysis of ATP to AMP and PP_i (Figure 5). Resynthesis of this AMP to ATP will require the energy equivalent of 2 ATP. Therefore, the net ATP production from one molecule of oleate would be $148 - 2 = 146$ molecules of ATP. Approximately 2,700 kcal of energy are contained in a mole of oleic acid. When oleate is oxidized in the muscle cell about 1,110 kcal (7.6 kcal/mol ATP $\times$ 146 mol ATP) are captured as high energy phosphate. The efficiency of energy transfer from oleate to ATP is thus about 41% (1,110/2,700). About 59% of the energy originally contained in the fatty acid molecules is lost as heat.

GLUCOSE METABOLISM

Though fat is the primary substrate in the normal muscle cell under conditions of rest or light to moderate activity and most of the required energy is derived from its oxidation, there is also a continuous catabolism of glucose. Like FFA, glucose is obtained from the circulating blood. Muscle cells may store glucose in the sarcoplasm as glycogen (Figure 3), which is simply a polymer of glucose molecules.

Unlike FFA molecules, glucose does not freely diffuse through the sarcolemma. In the absence of the pancreatic hormone insulin, glucose diffusion into muscle cells is greatly retarded. Because of lack of insulin, muscle tissue in diabetics is almost entirely dependent on non-carbohydrate sources for energy production. However, in the presence of insulin, glucose diffusion through the membrane is greatly facilitated, and adequate amounts may be obtained by the muscle cell.

After entering the fiber, glucose is immediately phosphorylated to glucose 6-phosphate in a reaction catalyzed by hexokinase (Figure 7). The phosphorylation is accomplished through transfer of the terminal phosphate of ATP to the glucose molecule. This reaction serves to trap glucose

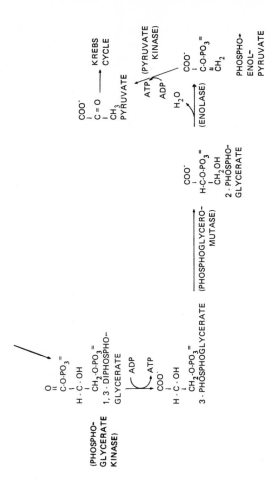

Figure 7. The Embden-Meyerhoff pathway.

in the cell, since glucose 6-phosphate cannot diffuse back through the membrane into the extracellular fluid. During periods of little or no muscle activity, most of this compound is converted to glycogen through a series of enzyme-catalyzed reactions. This polymerization of glucose produces relatively large granules of glycogen suitable for storage in the cell (Figure 3).

Aerobic Glycolysis

During muscle activity the glucose 6-phosphate may be directly metabolized for ATP production in a series of enzymatic reactions referred to as glycolysis (Embden-Meyerhoff pathway) (Figure 7). During the course of these reactions the 6-carbon glucose molecule is degraded to 2 3-carbon molecules. These molecules (glyceraldehyde 3-phosphate) are each oxidized (hydrogens removed) and the reducing equivalents transferred to the hydrogen carrier, NAD^+. The NADH delivers the reducing equivalents to the mitochondrion for ATP production under normal aerobic (with oxygen) conditions in the muscle cell (Figure 5). In 2 subsequent reactions in glycolysis, P_i is transferred from the carbohydrate molecules to ADP to form ATP. The end product of the aerobic glycolysis of glucose is pyruvate. Each glucose molecule is catabolized to 2 pyruvate molecules. The net reaction of the glycolytic oxidation of glucose to pyruvate is summarized in the following equation:

$$\text{Glucose} + 2NAD^+ + 2P_i + 2ADP \rightarrow 2 \text{ pyruvate} + 2 \text{ NADH} + 2H^+ + 2ATP$$

Phosphorylation at the substrate level produces a net of 2 molecules of ATP (early in the glycolytic sequence ATP is required for phosphorylation in the hexokinase and phosphofructokinase reactions), and the 2 pairs of hydrogens delivered to the respiratory chain result in the synthesis of 6 molecules of ATP. Thus, oxidation of one molecule of glucose to pyruvate allows the muscle cell to produce as many as 8 molecules of ATP.

Pyruvate may diffuse into the mitochondrion where it is converted to acetyl-CoA in a series of reactions catalyzed by the enzyme complex, pyruvate dehydrogenase (Figure 6). This complex catalyzes the removal of carbon dioxide from the pyruvate molecule and the subsequent condensation of the resulting 2-carbon fragment with Coenzyme A. During the conversion of pyruvate there is also a transfer of hydrogens to NAD^+.

Krebs Cycle

The acetyl-CoA molecules may then enter the Krebs cycle by condensing with oxalacetate, and the 2-carbon fragments become completely oxidized, as described in the section on fat catabolism in the muscle cell.

Thus, both carbohydrate and fat are degraded to the intermediate compound acetyl-CoA, and from that point their complete oxidation is accomplished in the same pathways. In glycolysis, one molecule of glucose provides only 2 molecules of acetyl-CoA, whereas β-oxidation of an oleic acid molecule produces 9. Oxidation of pyruvate is summarized in the following equation:

$$\text{Pyruvate} + 4NAD^+ + FAD + 3H_2O + ADP \rightarrow 3\ CO_2 +$$
$$4NADH + 4H^+ + FADH_2 + ATP$$

Oxidation of 2 molecules of pyruvate from 1 molecule of glucose in the Krebs cycle and the subsequent transfer of the resulting reducing equivalents to the respiratory chain produce 30 molecules of ATP, 2 at the substrate level in the Krebs cycle and 28 in the electron transport system.

If the energy stored with addition of the terminal phosphates in a mole of ATP is 7.6 kcal, the total energy captured as ATP from one mole of glucose is 7.6 kcal per mole × 38 moles, or 288.8 kcal. One mole of glucose is equivalent to 686 kcal, so approximately 42% of the energy of glucose is captured in ATP. The remaining 58% is released as heat. Therefore, the efficiency of ATP production from fats and carbohydrates is about the same under aerobic conditions.

Anaerobic Glycolysis

The generation of 38 molecules of ATP from 1 molecule of glucose is possible only if the muscle cell has an adequate supply of oxygen from the circulating blood. In the hypoxic condition the respiratory chain is limited by insufficient amounts of O_2. When hydrogen transfer to oxygen at the end of the electron transport system is retarded through lack of oxygen, the molecules in the chain become reduced and their acceptance of reducing equivalents from NADH or $FADH_2$ is impeded. In this situation, the hydrogen carriers in the mitochondrion exist in the reduced form (NADH and $FADH_2$). The Krebs cycle and glycolytic reactions that depend upon NAD^+ and FAD to accept hydrogens are therefore blocked and complete oxidation of substrates is restricted.

An extreme example of this situation occurs when a sprinter runs a 100-meter dash. The energy requirements of the exercising muscles are excessive and the fibers rapidly hydrolyze ATP for contractile energy. The resulting elevation in ADP activates the metabolic apparatus of the muscle cells in an attempt to maintain an adequate ATP concentration to support the exercise. However, in short, intense bursts of activity the circulating blood is not able to supply the muscle with adequate amounts of O_2 because of the lag times in elevation of cardiac output and the shifting of blood flow from other organs to the muscle, and because rapid and forceful contractions retard blood flow through the active muscle. Therefore, the oxidative processes in the mitochondrion cannot produce enough ATP to compensate for its rapid consumption in the contractile processes. Under these conditions the muscle is capable of producing limited quantities of ATP without a final reduction of oxygen in the electron transport system.

The primary substrate under these anaerobic conditions is glycogen, the stored glucose in the fiber. Ca^{2+} released by the sarcoplasmic reticulum to initiate contraction also activates the enzyme (phosphorylase) responsible for glycogenolysis (3). Thus, Ca^{2+} acts not only to enable the muscle fiber to contract, but also simultaneously to provide the cell with the nutrient energy source for ATP production. In 2 enzyme-catalyzed reactions, glycogen is degraded to glucose 6-phosphate, which is then metabolized in the glycolytic pathway (Figure 7). The reaction in which glyceraldehyde-3-phosphate is oxidized and the hydrogen accepted by NAD^+ however, is inhibited as the sarcoplasmic NAD^+ is converted to the reduced form (NADH). If the respiratory chain is not capable of receiving reducing equivalents from the sarcoplasm owing to low O_2 availability, all of the NAD^+ is converted to NADH and glycolysis is blocked at the dehydrogenase reaction. In hypoxic conditions, however, pyruvate may be reduced to lactate by transfer of hydrogens from NADH to pyruvate. This reaction is catalyzed by the enzyme lactate dehydrogenase. This allows glycolysis to proceed even though the mitochondria cannot accept all hydrogens from the NADH by replenishing cofactor (NAD^+) for the glyceraldehyde 3-phosphate dehydrogenase reaction. Every molecule of glucose (from glycogen) that is degraded to lactate in anaerobic glycolysis yields a net of 3 molecules of ATP (supply of glucose 6-phosphate from glycogen rather than from the blood bypasses the hexokinase reaction, which requires ATP). Though anaerobic glycolysis is inefficient compared with the complete oxidation of glucose (only 3 ATP as opposed to 38 ATP under aerobic conditions), these reactions are extremely rapid and enable the muscle cell to extend the time that exercise can be continued under hypoxic conditions.

Lactate produced in the muscle diffuses freely through the cell membrane into the blood so that tolerable levels of the acid metabolite are maintained in the intracellular environment up to very high work intensities. The circulating blood lactate may serve as a nutrient substrate in other organs, including the heart, where lactate is reconverted to pyruvate and completely oxidized to CO_2 and H_2O. In fact, skeletal muscle fibers have the enzymatic capacity to oxidize lactate, so that well-oxygenated fibers may catabolize this substrate during the exercise and all fibers may oxidize lactate following activity when blood flow supplies adequate oxygen (8).

It should be stressed that the normal muscle cell never relies entirely on anaerobic ATP production. The anaerobic process is initiated when aerobic metabolism is not sufficient to supply energy needs, but even under the most vigorous exercise conditions the cells receive some oxygen.

CONTROL OF SUBSTRATE AVAILABILITY TO THE MUSCLE CELL

In this discussion of metabolism the muscle fibers have been treated as a homogeneous population within the muscle, all having the same basic characteristics. In general terms this presentation reflects the actual situation, but it should be mentioned that human skeletal muscles are in fact composed of at least 2 distinct fiber types with different metabolic capacities. Thus, some human skeletal muscle fibers have relatively high concentrations of mitochondria and are better able to produce ATP aerobically, whereas others have a low oxidative capacity and must rely more on anaerobic energy production. Differences in the fiber types are discussed in detail in the preceding chapter.

In the resting condition and during low-intensity exercise, fatty acids are the primary fuel in skeletal muscle. However, as the exercise intensity increases, glycogen becomes more important as an energy source and it is possible that at very high power outputs the exercising muscle fibers catabolize only carbohydrate. Though the control mechanisms that determine the substrate to be used by the muscle cell under different conditions are complex, a major determining factor appears to be the availability of FFA to the cell. The uptake and combustion of FFA by muscle are proportional to their concentration in the blood (1). During exercise of low to moderate intensity, the utilization of FFA for ATP production parallels the elevation of FFA in the blood (4). As the power output of the muscle increases at higher exercise intensities, the role of carbohydrate becomes progressively more important (2). This relationship is dependent upon the blood supply to the exercising muscle. At rest and during light exercise, the blood flow is sufficient to supply both oxygen and FFA. At higher exercise intensities, glycogen catabolism increases owing to insufficient circulation to the muscle. In fact, the limiting factor in production of ATP as exercise becomes progressively more intense is probably the capacity of the circulation to deliver blood to the exercising muscle.

Levels of glucose and FFA in the blood vary little under normal conditions. Blood glucose concentration is about 100 mg per 100 ml of blood and plasma FFA levels are approximately 12 mg per 100 ml. Their concentrations in the blood are controlled by maintaining a balance between the release of the substances from their body storage sites and their uptake by peripheral tissues, including muscle. FFA are stored in adipose tissue as triglycerides. A triglyceride is composed of a glycerol backbone with 3 fatty acids attached to it. Fat tissue not only contains the excess fats consumed in the diet, but fatty acids formed from converted dietary carbohydrate and protein. Thus, regardless of whether the diet is composed of fat, protein, or carbohydrate, the excess is stored as triglycerides in the adipose tissue if caloric intake exceeds expenditure.

Several tissues in the body, particularly central nervous tissue and red blood cells, rely entirely on glucose for ATP production. Mechanisms that control substrate concentrations in the blood operate to insure adequate glucose supplies for these vital tissues. It is therefore of considerable functional significance that skeletal muscle, which comprises about 40% of the total body mass, can also oxidize fats for energy. FFA may be considered to have a "glucose-sparing" effect in skeletal muscle. It is known, for example, that FFA impair glucose metabolism in muscle fibers by indirectly inhibiting phosphofructokinase (a rate-limiting enzyme in glycolysis) activity (10). The hormone insulin plays a vital role in controlling substrate availability and metabolism in various body tissues, including skeletal muscle. Following a high carbohydrate meal, when blood glucose is elevated, insulin is released from the cells in the pancreas to promote glucose transport into peripheral tissues (e.g., skeletal muscle) and inhibit release of FFA from adipose tissue. Increased peripheral glucose uptake returns the blood concentration to normal levels and stimulates glucose metabolism. When blood glucose has declined to normal, insulin release from the pancreas diminishes, FFA concentration in the blood again rises, and fat becomes the dominant substrate in muscle tissue.

Net release of FFA from adipose tissue is controlled by factors other than insulin. Sympathetic nervous activity and release of catecholamines from the adrenal medulla both stimulate net release of FFA from fat stores. Also, a number of other hormones, e.g., growth hormone and ACTH, may cause plasma FFA levels to rise. Though hormonal and neural influences would tend to elevate FFA content in the blood during heavy exercise, its release is inhibited by lactate in the circulating blood (7). Thus, during high-intensity exercise, production of high levels of blood lactate by the active muscle prevents adipose tissue from releasing unnecessary amounts of FFA.

Blood glucose concentration in the post-absorptive state is maintained by the liver. Uptake of glucose by peripheral tissues is balanced by its release from this organ. The liver extracts glucose from the blood during the absorptive state, but it can also synthesize glucose from several other compounds obtained from the blood. The primary gluconeogenic substances are glycerol (which, along with FFA, is a product of triglyceride degradation), amino acids, and lactate. Glucose derived from gluconeogenesis or from the diet is stored as glycogen in the liver and is available for maintenance of blood glucose levels.

Though both muscle and liver maintain a glycogen reserve, the total energy stored as carbohydrate in the body is relatively small. In a 150-lb. man, approximately 1,100 kcal of energy are stored as glycogen. Normal blood glucose only contains about 20 kcal of energy. On the other hand, the same man would have about 45,000 kcal deposited as fat in adipose tissue. Though the amount of energy contained in the 2 stores varies considerably in different individuals, it is obvious that fat accumulations provide a considerably larger reservoir of potential energy for ATP production than carbohydrate stores.

It should also be emphasized that fat is a more efficient form of stored energy than carbohydrate. A unit weight of fat contains more than twice the energy as the same unit weight of carbohydrate (9.4 kcal and 4.2 kcal per gram for fat and carbohydrate, respectively). Moreover, glycogen storage is accompanied by increased H_2O retention by the cell, so fat constitutes a much "lighter" form of stored chemical energy.

It has been emphasized that under normal conditions in a healthy individual the major energy substrates in muscle are FFA and glucose. It was pointed out, however, that when blood lactate levels are elevated, the lactate may be oxidized by muscle cells for ATP production. This is particularly true in fibers with high mitochondrial content. Lactate concentration in the blood varies from about 1 mM at rest to as high as 20 mM during heavy exercise.

Ketone bodies constitute another form of substrate metabolized by skeletal muscle. These compounds appear in the blood in elevated concentrations when there is an abnormally high rate of FFA oxidation (e.g., in diabetes mellitus). In fact, there is evidence that ketone bodies may be metabolized preferentially by skeletal muscle when they are present in high plasma concentrations (12). However, under normal conditions keto acids do not contribute significantly to muscle fiber energy production.

LITERATURE CITED

1. Armstrong, D.T., R. Steele, N. Altszuler, A. Dunn, J.S. Bishop, and R.C. Debodo. 1961. Regulation of plasma free fatty acid turnover. Am. J. Physiol. 201:9–15.

2. Bergström, J., and E. Hultman. 1967. A study of the glycogen metabolism during exercise in man. Scand. J. Clin. Lab. Invest. 19:218–228.
3. Drummond, G.I., J.P. Harwood, and C.A. Powell. 1969. Studies on the activation of phosphorylase in skeletal muscle by contraction and by epinephrine. J. Biol. Chem. 244:4235–4240.
4. Hagenfeldt, L., and J. Wahren. 1971. Metabolism of free fatty acids and ketone bodies in skeletal muscle. *In* B. Pernow and B. Saltin (eds.), Muscle Metabolism During Exercise. Plenum, New York. pp. 153–163.
5. Hohorst, H.J., M. Reim, and H. Bartels. 1962. Studies on the creatine kinase equilibrium in muscle and the significance of ATP and ADP levels. Biochem. Biophys. Res. Comm. 7:142–146.
6. Hultman, E., J. Bergström, and N. McLennan Anderson. 1967. Breakdown and resynthesis of phosphoryl creatine and adenosine triphosphate in connection with muscular work in man. Scand. J. Clin. Lab. Invest. 19:56–66.
7. Issekutz, B., Jr., and H.I. Miller. 1962. Plasma free fatty acids during exercise and the effect of lactic acid. Proc. Soc. Exp. Biol. Med. 100:237–241.
8. Jorfeldt, L. 1971. Turnover of ^{14}C-L(+)-lactate in human skeletal muscle during exercise. *In* B. Pernow and B. Saltin (eds.), Muscle Metabolism During Exercise. Plenum, New York. pp. 409–417.
9. Mommaerts, W.F.H.M. 1969. Energetics of muscular contraction. Physiol. Rev. 49:427–508.
10. Scrutton, M.C., and M.F. Utter. 1968. The regulation of glycolysis and gluconeogenesis in animal tissues. Ann. Rev. Biochem. 37: 249–302.
11. Weber, A., and J.M. Murray. 1973. Molecular control mechanisms in muscle contraction. Physiol. Rev. 53:612–673.
12. Weiner, R., and J.J. Spitzer. 1973. Substrate utilization by myocardium and skeletal muscle in alloxan-diabetic dogs. Am. J. Physiol. 225:1288–1294.

PHYSIOLOGICAL RESPONSE TO PHYSICAL EXERCISE

Roger G. Soule

Response to physical exercise is reflected in all of the physiological systems of the human organism. Generally, physical exercise is thought of as using contractions in which the amount of force generated by the skeletal muscles is greater than the resistance against them, that is, shortening or concentric contractions. However, there are lengthening or eccentric contractions in which an external force overcomes the active muscle and the muscle is made to lengthen. Also, there are isometric contractions in which the force generated by the muscle is equal to the resistance and there is no movement.

Many factors affect the ability of an individual to perform exercise. Two of a general overriding concern are age and sex. Then, environmental stresses such as altitude, hyperbaric conditions, heat, and cold influence performance. Within the boundaries of the above, other factors are operating: acclimatization to the stress, training, and detraining programs. Further, the intensity and duration of exercise influences the ability to perform. Body position and the characteristics of the individual muscle groups are also reflected in the execution of the exercise, as well as factors playing a part in affecting physiological function of the systems, such as oxygen transport, circulation, pulmonary action, and cardiac performance and metabolism, to mention a few.

UTILIZATION OF OXYGEN

The first concept to be considered is oxygen utilization, determined and expressed as oxygen uptake (V_{O_2}). The energy yield from every liter of

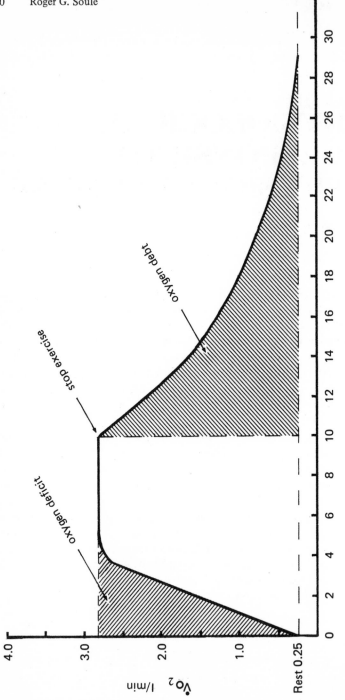

Figure 1. Pattern of oxygen consumption during and after physical exercise involving concentric muscle contractions and characterized as of moderate intensity.

oxygen consumed by the body ranges from a low of 4.7 kcal/l with pure fat as the energy-yielding substrate, to a high of 5.05 kcal/l if the energy source is carbohydrate. The kcal yield per liter of oxygen uptake is taken to be 4.85 if the person is utilizing an average mixed diet as the substrate pool. This condition would produce an R.Q. (respiratory quotient) value of 0.85. For a simple calculation of energy costs a value of 5.0 kcal/l of oxygen utilized is acceptable.

In Figure 1 the traditional $\dot{V}O_2$ curve for a moderate level of exercise is shown. Within the first 3–4 minutes, (or sooner at certain intensities of exercise) the ability to take up oxygen in sufficient quantity to meet the metabolic demand of the skeletal muscle tissues is attained. Thereafter, if the exercise is of moderate intensity, the need and the availability of oxygen are balanced and the so-called "steady-state" oxygen uptake is observed. In Figure 2 it is apparent that, as the exercise intensity varies, the oxygen need of the tissues changes. The values shown in the figure should not be taken as absolute, but only to approximate an average oxygen need for a given exercise intensity. The greater the exercise intensity the greater will be the metabolic demands of the tissues for oxygen, especially in the skeletal muscle cells, up to the limits of the system (19). The greatest amount of oxygen that can be taken up and used by the body for a given unit of time has been termed the maximal oxygen uptake ($\dot{V}O_2$ max) or aerobic capacity.

ANAEROBIC METABOLISM

As the need or demand for oxygen goes beyond the maximal delivery capability, the exercise may be continued only through the utilization of anaerobic metabolic mechanisms. Anaerobic metabolism allows for the yielding of energy from carbohydrate stores without the immediate availability of adequate volumes of oxygen. When this is the case, the end product of the energy release of carbohydrate will yield lactate. It is important to note that the property of the lactate molecule to accept H^+ is an enabling mechanism for the continuance of exercise. However, there may be a time during exercise when the depletion of energy substrates of the accumulation of lacate could be the causative factor for stopping exercise.

EXERCISE WITH ECCENTRIC AND ISOMETRIC CONTRACTIONS

The availability of oxygen (either immediately or ultimately) is thus essential in order to perform exercise using concentric skeletal muscle contractions. At this point, a brief look at oxygen uptake in exercise using

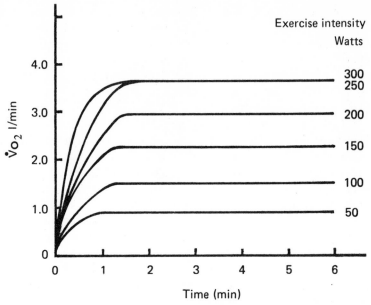

Figure 2. Relationship of oxygen uptake to various exercise intensities involving concentric muscle contractions. Note there is no additional increase in oxygen uptake with further increase in exercise intensity once maximal oxygen uptake is reached.

eccentric and isometric contractions is in order. In Figure 3 data are presented showing a comparison of oxygen uptake during exercise of concentric versus eccentric contractions. These data are representative of the differences usually observed, in that exercise of approximately three times the intensity was required to cause a comparable oxygen uptake using eccentric contractions compared to concentric. The relationship may show some variations under varying conditions (e.g., faster or slower rpm) but the general observation of much lower oxygen cost for the development of tension with eccentric contractions does not change.

Other considerations should be of concern in the comparison of cycle ergometer exercise of concentric and eccentric contractions. Data exhibited in Figure 4 present examples of two of these other concerns: the interrelated influences of pedal frequency and exercise intensity on the oxygen cost of exercise. Oxygen uptake values are presented for a range of exercise intensities performed at three pedal frequencies. It is apparent that the oxygen uptake is greater for the concentric exercise at all comparable pedal frequencies and intensities. It should be noted that the highest pedal frequency, 100 rpm, demonstrated the highest net efficiency

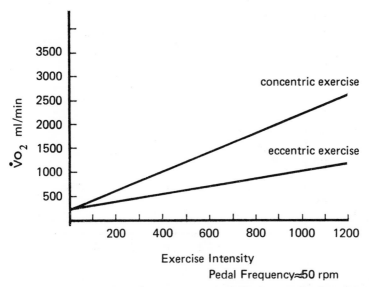

Figure 3. Relationship of steady-state oxygen uptake to exercise intensity per-formed with eccentric as compared with concentric muscle contractions. The pedal frequency is approximately 50 rpm. (Adapted from Asmussen, E. 1952. Acta Physiologica Scandinavica 28:364–382.)

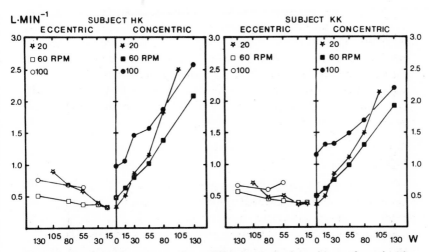

Figure 4. Steady-state oxygen uptake at different exercise intensities performed with concentric and eccentric muscle contractions at 3 pedal frequencies. (Taken from Knuttgen, H.G. 1971. Medicine and Science in Sports 3:1–5.)

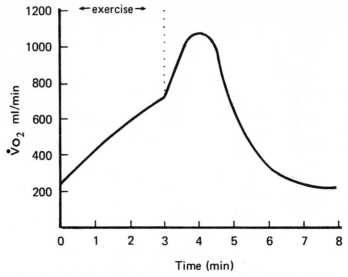

Figure 5. Characteristic curve of oxygen uptake during and after high intensity isometric leg exercise involving sustained muscle contractions.

when calculated over and above free wheeling cost, as indicated by the slope of the lines representing $\dot{V}O_2$ versus intensity. The lowest pedal frequency evidenced the lowest slope and therefore the lowest efficiency.

A brief look at oxygen uptake during an isometric contraction completes this consideration. The general response to moderate and heavy exercise is demonstrated in Figure 5. While an isometric contraction is maintained, there is gradual increase in oxygen uptake as energy is required for the skeletal muscle tissue's attempt to shorten. As relaxation occurs, there is an accompanying increase in blood flow to the muscles that results in an increased availability of oxygen and a concurrent marked increase in oxygen uptake.

SUBSTRATE UTILIZATION

Following this discussion of oxygen utilization, it is logical to consider the foodstuffs or substrates involved in the energy release to which the oxygen uptake is related during the exercise. It is well known that the major energy contributors, even at rest, are fats and carbohydrates. The role of protein seems to be primarily related to muscle metabolism, with a minimal daily intake, approximately 60 g/day, needed for this purpose.

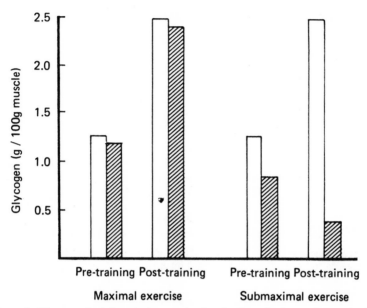

Figure 6. Glycogen depletion during maximal and submaximal exercise employing concentric muscle contractions. Rest, □; Fatigue, ▨. (Adapted from Taylor, A.W. 1971. Medicine and Science in Sports 3:75–78.)

During exercise, the protein involvement as an energy source is considered to be negligible. For the present discussion nonprotein data will be considered. At rest, approximately 55% of the energy is coming from fat metabolism and the remainder from carbohydrate. The interaction of these two substrates as exercise is started in quite interesting and predictable. As exercise is begun and the intensity is increased (the higher the percent of $\dot{V}O_2$ max), the greater the contribution the carbohydrate stores of glycogen will make. High intensity exercise, and thus limited in time of performance, uses primarily glycogen as a substrate. During long-term exercise of moderate intensity (e.g., below 75% $\dot{V}O_2$ max) the involvement of the fat stores appears to be much greater.

First, the data of Figure 6 will be considered. It may be observed from the modified data of Taylor et al. (21) that, as previously mentioned, although carbohydrate is the primary energy source during high intensity exhaustive exercise, the depletion of the glycogen stores is minimal in exhaustive exercise; that is, the depletion of the glycogen stores is limited in untrained and trained subjects (the duration of exercise is so short and the total energy requirement to exhaustion is really quite small, 5–7 g of

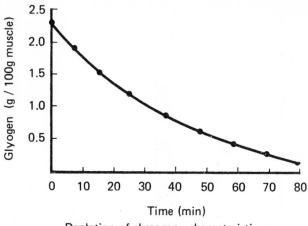

Depletion of glycogen - characteristic curve

Figure 7. Characteristic pattern of glycogen depletion from thigh muscle during long-lasting concentric leg exercise of high intensity.

glycogen) (*21*). When a subject exercises at a lower intensity (e.g. 40–80% of $\dot{V}O_2$ max), and consequently continues for a much longer time before exhaustion, the minute by minute percentage involvement of glycogen becomes less. However, the total use of glycogen is greater because the time is so much longer, perhaps 90 min versus 5–6 min. The glycogen reserves of muscle and liver are used, and, at some point, if exercise is continued long enough, are said to be, practically speaking, depleted.

The general configuration of the relationship of glycogen depletion with time as related to exercise intensity is shown in Figure 7, a composite of several studies (*4, 5, 7, 9, 21*). The assumption is usually made that the depletion of the muscle glycogen reserves and the cessation of exercise occur at the same time; at least subjects have not demonstrated an ability to exercise after the glycogen levels were very low. This occurence seems to be true for individuals at many levels of training, from sedentary to and including well-trained individuals, with perhaps the well trained able to deplete to a slightly greater degree (*7, 20, 21*). If the initial muscle glycogen levels were elevated as a result of training and diet control, it appears that the length of time to exhaustion is lengthened (*4, 5, 6, 8*). From this discussion it is apparent that involvement of the glycogen stores is important, especially during high intensity short-term and moderate intensity long-term exercise. Recent data have also indicated an importance of glycogen stores for stop-go types of anaerobic exercise such as

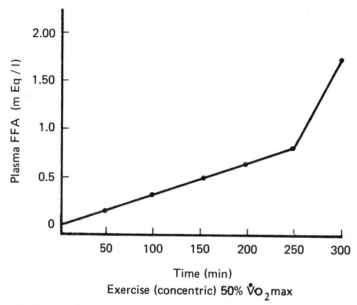

Figure 8. Plasma free fatty acid concentration during exercise involving concentric contractions at 50% of aerobic power capacity. (Adapted from Pruett, E.D.R. 1970. Journal of Applied Physiology 29:809–815.)

soccer (20). Whether or not the depletion of the glycogen from the muscle is the actual cause of the person stopping exercise has not been conclusively demonstrated.

During exercise of moderate intensity and of greater than 30 min duration the involvement of fat reserves is greatly increased. One indication of fat store involvement is the level of plasma free fatty acids (FFA).

Figure 8 shows the general FFA level in plasma with exercise at 50% of $\dot{V}O_2$ max plotted against time. These data show that the involvement of FFA does become greater as time passes. The involvement of fats with long-term exercise has been well documented (1, 5, 6, 8, 10, 11, 12, 13, 16).

The interaction of fats and carbohydrates during exercise shown in Figure 9 indicates that, as exercise intensity is increased, carbohydrate involvement is increased, while the remaining energy is derived from fat.

The discussion thus far has not pointed to the more immediate energy stores, the high-energy phosphates. Adenosine triphosphate (ATP), creatine phosphate (CP), and lactate concentrations in muscle have been studied during concentric and eccentric exercise (6, 8, 15). These data are summarized in Figure 10. Eccentric exercise does not result in any signifi-

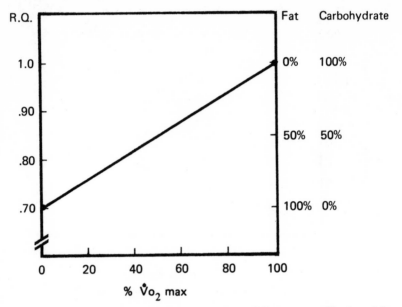

Figure 9. Relationships among respiratory quotient (RQ), percent utilization of fat vs. carbohydrate, and exercise intensity relative to aerobic power capacity.

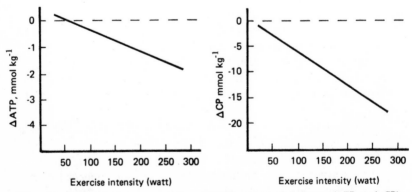

Figure 10. Depletion in concentration of high-energy phosphates (ATP and CP) during steady-state exercise involving concentric contractions. (Taken from Knutt-gen, H.G., and B. Saltin. 1972. Journal of Applied Physiology 32:690–694.)

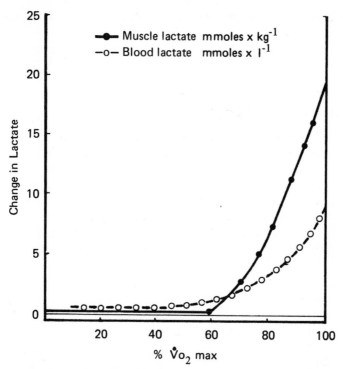

Figure 11. Relationship of muscle and blood lactate concentration to exercise involving concentric (closed symbols) and eccentric contractions (open symbols). (Taken from Knuttgen, H.G., and B. Saltin. 1972. Journal of Applied Physiology 32: 690–694.)

cant changes in muscles concentration of ATP or CP or to increases in lactate at a $\dot{V}O_2$ of approximately 1.0 l/m (an exercise intensity of approximately 200 W). During the period of exercise (which lasted approximately 30 min), the accumulation of lactate in the exercising muscle, as measured from the venous blood, did not differ significantly from rest.

In short-term concentric exercise at higher intensities, the increase in lactate is more dramatic in the exercising skeletal muscle than in the blood. This response is apparent in Figure 11, where four-minute exercise data are shown. As the exercise intensity becomes closer and closer to the $\dot{V}O_2$ max value, the level of lactate becomes higher in both muscle and blood, pointing to the increased anaerobic involvement in the exercise.

Although there does not appear to be a balance between the muscle and the blood lactate during such exercise, this does not mean that under certain steady-state conditions these values could not attain equilibrium, However, it should be reiterated at this point that it is the interaction of fats and carbohydrates (see Figure 9), that provide the energy for ATP synthesis for all intensities of exercise.

PULMONARY VENTILATION

Under the various conditions for exercise the ventilative response is in direct proportion to the intensity of the exercise. The magnitude of the response will differ among the conditions because of the quantitative relationship between ventilation and oxygen uptake. A comparison of minute volume of expired air ($\dot{V}e$) in arm versus leg exercise with concentric contractions is shown in Figure 12. A description of the response may be generalized by saying the ventilation closely follows that of the $\dot{V}O_2$ during exercise of concentric, eccentric, and isometric exercise up through

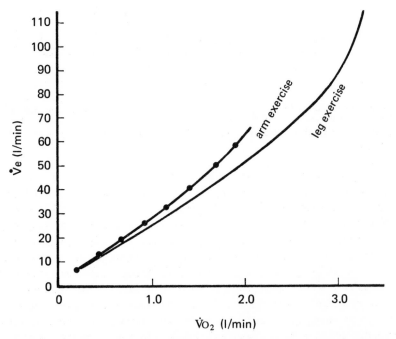

Figure 12. Pulmonary ventilation relative to steady-state oxygen uptake for arm vs. leg exercise involving concentric contractions. (Adapted from Vokac, Z., et al. 1975. Journal of Applied Physiology 39:1, 54–59.)

moderate levels of exercise intensity. At high exercise intensities the responses do not follow each other as closely (3, 22).

CIRCULATION

As a final consideration of the general response to exercise, the common circulatory responses should be discussed. The relationships among cardiac output, oxygen uptake, and the arterial and venous oxygen concentrations are represented as follows:

$$\dot{Q} = \frac{\dot{V}O_2}{aO_2 - \bar{v}O_2}$$

Where: $\dot{Q}$ = Cardiac output (l/min of blood)
$\dot{V}O_2$ = Oxygen consumption (ml of O_2/min)
aO_2 = Arterial concentration of oxygen (approximately 20 vol%)
$\bar{v}O_2$ = Mixed venous concentration of oxygen (measured value)

Transformation of the equation and substitution of knowns ($\dot{Q}$ = heart rate (HR) times strokes volume (SV)) the equation becomes:

$$\dot{V}O_2 = HR \times SV \times (aO_2 - \bar{v}O_2)$$

As exercise begins, the HR, SV and arterial-venous oxygen differences all increase in direct proportion as the intensity is increased, continuing up to maximum exercise levels. However, as observed in Figure 13, stroke volume reaches 100% value at approximately 40% of the $\dot{V}O_2$ max value, while the heart rate response continues to increase up to exercise intensities resulting in $\dot{V}O_2$ near maximal.

It appears the percent of $\dot{V}O_2$ max is an important consideration for heart rate as well as stroke volume, as indicated in Figure 14. The heart rate response is shown to follow the same pattern for eccentric as well as concentric contractions (Figure 13). The oxygen uptake response elicits a similar heart rate response whether the exercise is with concentric or eccentric contractions. However, the exercise intensity needed to elicit an identical heart rate is, as observed with $\dot{V}O_2$, much higher with eccentric contractions than with concentric.

The relationships of a − $\bar{v}$ oxygen difference and cardiac output to oxygen uptake are demonstrated in Figure 15. Cardiac output demonstrates increases to maximal values at or near $\dot{V}O_2$ max (18). A similar observation can be made for a − $\bar{v}$ oxygen difference. It has been shown that under certain conditions, small increases in oxygen uptake can be

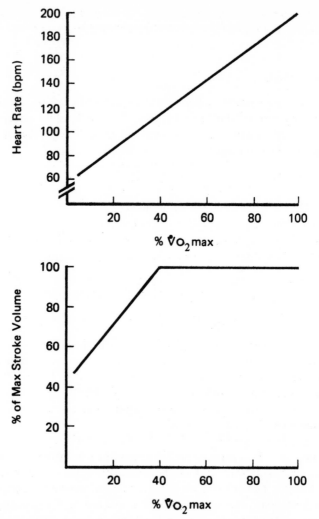

Figure 13. Heart rate (bpm = beats per min) and stroke volume relative to steady-state oxygen uptake for leg exercise involving concentric contractions.

achieved at intensities above those eliciting $\dot{Q}$ max, as a result of small additional increases in a $-\bar{v}O_2$ difference.

Summarizing cardiac considerations during exercise: as the oxygen needs of the tissues increase as a result of the exercise intensity, the cardiac components, both heart rate and stroke volume, increase up to

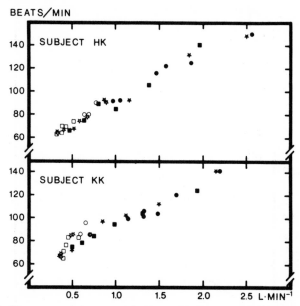

BEATS/MIN

Figure 14. Heart rate relative to steady-state oxygen uptake during cycling exercise involving concentric (closed symbols) and eccentric contractions (open symbols). (From Knuttgen, H.G., et al. 1971. Medicine and Science in Sports, 3:1–5.)

maximum values. During the exercise, the arterial venous oxygen difference in the exercising muscles also increases to maximum values. When each of the parameters mentioned is at maximum value, further increases in exercise intensity may be accomplished for short time periods, 1–3–5 min, only through the use of anaerobic metabolic mechanisms.

CONCLUSION

A generalized but brief look has been taken at the physiological response to exercise in humans. There are many individual differences in response and the magnitude of the response may be related to the state of training. However, the direction of the response for each of the systems considered will be in the same direction regardless of the level of training. There are other magnitude of response differences when performing exercise using concentric, eccentric, or isometric skeletal muscle contractions. Other physiological parameters that respond to exercise that have not been mentioned here include: neurological, enzymatic, and hormonal factors. In

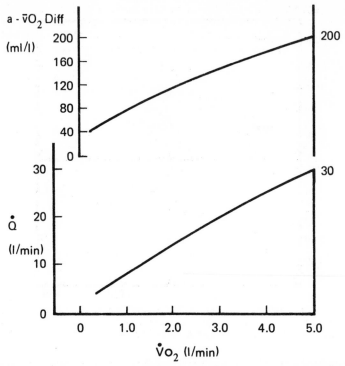

Figure 15. Arterio-venous oxygen difference and minute volume of cardiac output relative to steady-state of oxygen uptake during exercise with concentric muscle contractions. (Adapted from Rowell, L.B. 1974. Physiological Reviews 54:75–79.)

summary, a single exercise session of any intensity elicits physiological responses from people no matter what their level of physical training. The degree to which training will enhance or diminish these responses will be considered in the following chapter, "Development of Muscular Strength and Endurance."

LITERATURE CITED

1. Armstrong, D.T., R. Steele, N. Altszuler, A. Dunn, J.S. Bishop and C. DeBodo. 1961. Regulation of plasma free fatty acid turnover. Am. J. Physiol. 201:9–15.
2. Asmussen, E. 1952. Positive and negative muscular work. Acta Physiol. Scand. 28:364–382.

3. Åstrand, P.O., and K. Rodahl. 1970. Textbook of Work Physiology. McGraw-Hill Book Company, New York.
4. Bergström, J., and E. Hultman. 1966. Muscle glycogen synthesis after exercise: An enhancing factor localized to the muscle cells in man. Nature 210:309.
5. Bergström, J., L. Hermansen, E. Hultman, and B. Saltin. 1967. Diet, muscle glycogen, and physical performance. Acta Physiol. Scand. 71:140–150.
6. Fröberg, S.O., and F. Massfeldt. 1971. Effect of prolonged strenuous exercise on the concentration of triglycerides, phospholipids and glycogen in muscle of man. Acta Physiol. Scand. 82:167–171.
7. Gollnick, P.D., R.B. Armstrong, C.W. Saubert IV, R.C. Shepherd, and B. Saltin. 1973. Glycogen depletion patterns in human skeletal muscle fibers after exhausting exercise. J. Appl. Physiol. 34: 615–618.
8. Gollnick, P.D., R.G. Soule, A.W. Taylor, C. Williams, and C.D. Ianuzzo. 1970. Exercise-induced glycogenolysis and lipolysis in the rat: Hormonal influence. Am. J. Physiol. 219:729–733.
9. Hermansen, L., E. Hultman, and B. Saltin. 1967. Muscle glycogen during prolonged severe exercise. Acta Physiol. Scand. 71:129–139.
10. Issekutz, B., Jr., H.I. Miller, and K. Rodahl. 1963. Effects of exercise on FFA metabolism of pancreatectomized dogs. Am. J. Physiol. 205:645–650.
11. Karlsson, J., S. Rosell, and B. Saltin. 1972. Carbohydrate and fat metabolism in contracting canine skeletal muscle. Pflugers Arch. 331:57–69.
12. Keul, J. 1973. The relationship between circulation and metabolism during exercise. Med. Sci. Sports 5:209–219.
13. Keul, J., E. Doll, and D. Keppler. 1972. Energy metabolism of human muscle, S. Karger, Basel.
14. Knuttgen, H.G., F. Bonde-Petersen, and K. Klausen. 1971. Oxygen uptake and heart rate responses to exercise performed with concentric and eccentric muscle contractions. Med. Sci. Sports 3:1–5.
15. Knuttgen, H.G., and B. Saltin. 1972. Muscle metabolites and oxygen uptake in short-term submaximal exercise in man. J. Appl. Physiol. 32(5):690–694.
16. Pruett, E.D.R. 1970. FFA mobilization during and after prolonged severe muscular work in men. J. Appl. Physiol. 29(6):809–815.
17. Pruett, E.D.R. 1970. Glucose and insulin during prolonged work stress in men living on different diets. J. Appl. Physiol. 28(2):199–208.
18. Rowell, L.B. 1974. Human cardiovascular adjustments to exercise and thermal stress. Physiol. Rev. 54:75–159.
19. Saltin, B., and P.O. Åstrand. 1967. Maximal oxygen uptake in athletes. J. Appl. Physiol. 23:353–358.
20. Saltin, B. 1973. Metabolic fundamentals in exercise. Med. Sci. Sports 5:137–146.

21. Taylor, A.W., R. Lappage, and S. Rao. 1971. Skeletal muscle glycogen stores after submaximal and maximal work. Med. Sci. Sports. 3: 75–78.

22. Vocac, Z., H. Bell, E. Bautz-Holter, and K. Rodahl. 1975. Oxygen uptake–heart rate relationship in leg and arm exercise, sitting and standing. J. Appl. Physiol. 39:54–59.

Development of Muscular Strength and Endurance

Howard G. Knuttgen

CONTRACTION CHARACTERISTICS OF ISOLATED MUSCLE

For an understanding of the strength and endurance capabilities of a person engaged in physical exercise, an examination of the characteristics of an isolated muscle provides a good starting point. It has already been pointed out that, when stimulated muscle attempts to shorten, the external resistance will determine whether the muscle overcomes the resistance (concentric contraction), is matched by the resistance (isometric contraction), or is overcome by the resistance (eccentric contraction).

Force versus Length Relationships

Figure 1 presents the results of a series of experiments in which isolated muscle is both stretched without innervation (passive stretching) and also subjected to maximal stimulation at various lengths. On the abscissa, R indicates the resting length that the muscle would assume when no efferent impulses were being received. Moving along the abscissa to the right is indicative of increased length or stretching and to the left is indicative of decreased length (both indicated in arbitrary units).

If a resting muscle is passively stretched, a force is developed owing to the elastic qualities of the muscle alone (the parallel elastic component). The greater the degree of stretch, the greater the force becomes as the muscle attempts to resume resting length. The relation-

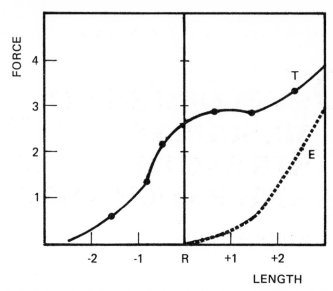

Figure 1. Relationship of force (tension) to length for an isolated skeletal muscle preparation. Curve designated as *E* is for elastic force (parallel elastic component) developed when unstimulated muscle is stretched from resting length (*R* on abscissa). Curve designated as *T* is total force (contractile force plus elastic force) for muscle stimulated maximally in isometric contractions at various lengths. To the right (+) on the abscissa indicates lengths greater than resting while to the left (−) indicates lengths less than resting.

ship of force to length for this condition is curvilinear and is shown in Figure 1 by the broken line identified as *E* (for "elastic"). Elastic force terminates at resting length and, therefore, no relationship exists to the left of *R* on the abscissa.

If the muscle is then subjected to a series of experiments in which the length is first established (and maintained) before a maximal tetanic stimulation, the relationship of length to force of isometric contraction is established. As the degree of stimulation is always maximal, the force of contraction will be maximal for each condition of length.

The results of such experiments are shown as the filled circle symbols and the relationship of length to isometric contraction force established by the solid line (identified as *T* for Total Force). The following observations can be made:

1. The total force generated is greater when a muscle is in a stretched condition than in a shorter resting condition.
2. The shorter the length of the muscle from the resting condition the less the force developed during isometric contraction.

3. In general, the greater the length of the muscle from the resting condition the greater the total force developed during isometric contraction.

The relationship described has been designated as that of Total Force to muscle length and the curve identified as T. This is because the force developed at greater-than-resting lengths (to the right of R) is the sum total of the contractile force (generated in the sarcomeres) *plus* the elastic force already described. As the parallel elastic component is not active at less than resting lengths, the total force generated is due to the contractile elements. In order to determine the force generated by the contractile elements at any length greater than resting, the elastic force would be subtracted from the total force. In Figure 1, this would be the distance between curves E and T.

Force versus Velocity Relationship

All of the experiments in Figure 1 were performed at predetermined lengths and, therefore, the contractions were isometric. The next relationship to be examined is when a muscle (in maximal tetanic stimulation) is allowed to shorten at different velocities or is forcibly stretched at different velocities.

In Figure 2, the results of such experiments are presented. The 0 on the abscissa indicates zero velocity or the isometric condition. To the right, the arbitrary units indicate velocity of eccentric contractions (the higher the positive number the greater the velocity). To the left, the arbitrary negative numbers indicate comparative velocities of concentric contractions. The muscle is always stimulated maximally, so the recorded force is recorded as maximal force (and represents total force). The following observations can be made:

1. Forces of concentric contractions of any and all velocities are less than forces generated under the isometric and eccentric conditions.
2. The greater the velocity of a concentric contraction the less the external force generated.
3. Forces of lengthening contractions of any and all velocities are greater than the isometric and concentric maxima.
4. The faster a lengthening contraction the greater the force (up to very high velocities where a leveling off occurs).

The forces developed in the series of experiments described were recorded in each case at a predetermined length of the muscle. If such determinations were at a different length, the magnitude of the forces

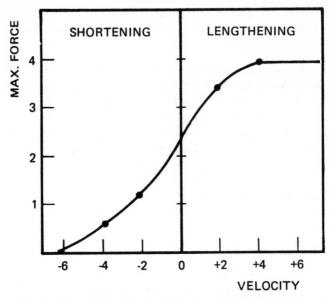

Figure 2. Relationship of force to velocity for an isolated muscle preparation under maximal stimulation. From left to right on the abscissa are rapid concentric (shortening) contraction, slow shortening contraction, isometric contraction (0), slow eccentric (lengthening) contraction, and rapid eccentric contraction.

recorded would change but the general configuration of the curve would remain unchanged.

Relating the observations for Figure 2 to the results of the initial figure, certain additional observations can be added to Figure 1. If the forces recorded by a concentrically contracting muscle (at any velocity) are drawn in at the various length changes the muscle passes through, all forces would fall under the line designating total isometric force (less force is generated in concentric than isometric contraction) and the faster the velocity of concentric contraction the further below the total force line as shown in Figure 1. Conversely, if the forces recorded during an eccentric contraction were added to Figure 1, the forces would fall above the isometric force line. The faster the velocity of the eccentric contraction the further above the line.

FORCE POTENTIALS IN HUMAN MOVEMENT

The question can now be raised as to the similarity of muscle performance in the human to the observations on the isolated muscle prepa-

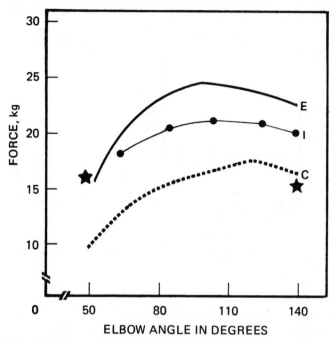

Figure 3. Relationship of maximal force of human elbow flexor muscles to elbow position for three types of contraction: eccentric (*E*), isometric (*I*), and concentric (*C*). (Figure adapted from Singh and Karpovich (*39*).)

rations. Two studies (*2, 39*) provide the answer to this question very nicely and results of these studies are presented in Figures 3 and 4. All of the results presented are obtained for the elbow flexor muscles with the action of flexion involved in the concentric contractions and with the action of elbow extension when the flexors are being forcibly overcome for eccentric contraction. All contractions represent maximal voluntary force and could be termed 1 Repetition Maximum (1 RM). (1 RM or 1 Repetition Maximum: a maximal voluntary contraction which, due to its exhaustive intensity, cannot be followed by a second repetition (*6*).)

In Figure 3, the subject is attached to a motor-driven lever that can record force while in motion or when stopped at any angle. It is evident that, at any elbow angle, eccentric contraction gives the greatest force, concentric the lowest, and isometric is intermediate (a single velocity was employed for the concentric and eccentric experiments). The lower forces at the extremities of each curve represent a

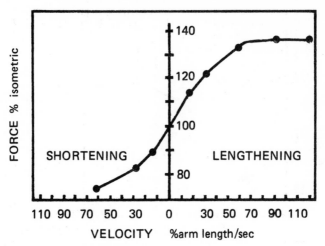

Figure 4. Relationship of maximal force of human elbow flexor muscles to velocity. Velocity on abscissa is designated as percent of arm length per second. (Figure adapted from E. Asmussen et al. (2).)

combination of diminished mechanical advantage at these angles and disadvantageous lengths in the muscles' force-length relationships.

In Figure 4, the results are presented for experiments conducted with human subjects at a wide range of velocities on a similar device. The maximal forces recorded at a designated elbow angle result in a curve configuration that appears identical to Figure 2.

FUNCTIONAL CAPACITIES OF THE EXERCISING HUMAN

All of the data presented thus far represent muscular efforts that could not be immediately repeated and, therefore, the forces recorded for each represent what could be termed 1 Repetition Maximum. We shall now examine the relationship of exercise involving the full range of force expression to a person's ability to repeat the particular movement or activity.

The results of experiments performed with two ergometers on a healthy, adult subject are presented in Figure 5. In the left portion, a finger ergograph was employed for the activity of the third digit in a flexing movement. In the right portion, a cycle ergometer was used for cycling exercise for the legs. Note that in both cases the activity for the muscles involves almost exclusively concentric contractions.

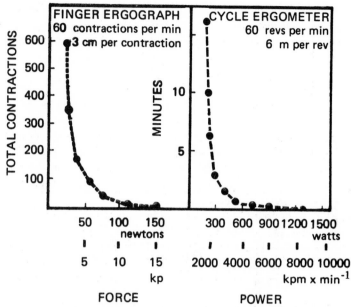

Figure 5. *Left panel:* Relationship of endurance (as total contractions) of re-peated flexion of third digit to effective force of contraction. *Right panel:* Rela-tionship of endurance (as minutes of fatigue) of cycle ergometer exercise to ex-ternal power production. In both panels, the intercept with the abscissa represents the exercise intensity for which the maneuver could be performed only once (and, therefore, the strength of the concentric movement). In both panels, endurance could be presented as either total contractions or minutes to fatigue and, as the contraction rate and velocity are designated, either abscissa could be designated as force (per individual repetition) or power (work per unit time).

Finger Ergograph Exercise

All exercise is being performed with flexion of the 3rd digit at a rate of 60 contractions per min. The force (as determined by the resis-tance) is expressed through 3 cm each contraction. If the action of the finger returning to the starting point after each contraction is ig-nored, the force of the contractions is expressed through 180 cm per min (which can be used as an index of velocity of the activity).

At a resistance of 150 N (or 15 kiloponds), the muscles can per-form the flexion but one time. This is the 1 Repetition Maximum (1 RM) and can be designated the strength of the movement. At 50% of the maximum (resistance of 75 N) the person can continue the activity for 50 contractions or 50 sec. At 15% of the maximum, the activity can be sustained for 600 contractions for 10 min. As the endurance curve becomes asymptotic below this level, lower intensities could be continued indefinitely.

Cycle Ergometer Exercise

All cycling exercise is being performed in the example at 60 pedal revolutions per minute (60 rpm) and, therefore, the velocity is constant. The flywheel turns 6 m per pedal revolution so that its velocity is 360 m per min under all conditions. The greatest power for this person was 1,300 W (or 8,000 kilopond-meters/min). This was something the subject could perform for only one revolution (one push by each leg) and, therefore, represents a 1 RM.

At 200 W or lower, the person could sustain the power output for relatively long periods of time (15 min and longer). At 100 W or lower, the exercise could be maintained indefinitely.

A person's maximal oxygen uptake ($\dot{V}O_2$ max) is usually elicited in exercise of this type, which causes fatigue in somewhere between 3 and 10 min. For this person, this would involve exercise intensities (power outputs) in the range of 240 to 300 W. Relating this power to that mentioned for the 1 RM (which could be accepted as the *strength* of a leg thrust), the average force being produced by each leg in order to elicit the person's maximal oxygen uptake amounts to 25% or less of the 1 RM.

Endurance and Fatigue

The physiological capacities that determine the configuration of the curves are probably as follows:

1. The intercept with the abscissa (the 1 RM, or strength) is determined by the cross-sectional area of the muscles involved.
2. The horizontal portion of the curve is determined predominantly by the capacity of the anaerobic energy release processes.
3. The vertical portion of the curve is determined by the aerobic energe release capacity as dominated by the delivery of oxygen to the muscles by the circulatory system.
4. The portion of greatest curvilinearity is related to a combination of aerobic and anaerobic power capacities.

At the 1 RM level, we might look to the central nervous system, the myoneural junction, or the excitation mechanisms within the muscle cells for why the exertion can't be repeated (i.e., why "fatigue" occurs). At very high power levels, at which contractions can be repeated up to 10 times, we might look for some combination of fatigue of excitation mechanisms and/or depletion of high-energy phosphate at the sites of contractile activity (the myofilaments).

At sustained high power levels, generally described as anaerobic in nature, (e.g., 10 sec to 100 sec duration), certain metabolic factors can be added: high-energy phosphate depletion owing to the inability of glycolysis to maintain sufficient ATP resynthesis and/or the deleterious effects of local lactate or hydrogen ion accumulation on the cellular processes.

At activity levels that can be maintained for 3 to 10 min, we would hypothesize that the endurance is limited by a combination of anaerobic and aerobic factors; the lower the exercise intensities or power demands the more important is the role of oxygen. While controversy exists over the importance of oxygen delivery (circulatory limitation) versus oxygen utilization (cellular metabolic limitation) under various conditions, there is little doubt that the inability of the mechanisms of oxidative phosphorylation (Krebs cycle and electron transport system) to resynthesize ATP determines endurance in the upper part of this middle range (e.g., 5 min to as long as 30 min). The increases in concentration of lactate and hydrogen ions are quite pronounced in the shorter durations and could constitute factors of importance for limiting the performance of the exercising muscle (23).

At exercise intensities that can be maintained for extended periods (1 to 2 hr), depletion of endogenous glycogen (stored in the muscle cells themselves) is the most likely factor (21). Because the uptake rate of glucose from the blood is limited, depletion of the glycogen curtails both glycolytic phosphorylation and the availability of carbohydrate-provided substrate (pyruvate) for the Krebs cycle.

It should be emphasized that most of the above information has been obtained in exercise involving large portions of the body musculature (cycle ergometer exercise and treadmill running). The statements made are probably applicable to both situations, with one major exception. Maximal cardiac output (which will be discussed under the section "Conditioning Programs for Aerobic Power Capacity") is of great importance for the cycle ergometer exercise but not related to the physiological factors involved in finger exercise.

Limitations of Figure 5

The relationships presented in Figure 5 demonstrate vividly that physical performance is quite different at the various power levels of which the person is capable. At the same time, the interrelationship of muscle bulk, anaerobic power, and aerobic power is demonstrated.

Before the examples become accepted for more than they deserve, certain limitations and precautions should be enumerated:

1. The intercepts identified as the person's strengths for the movements are actually only for the concentric condition. The isometric strengths should be greater and lie further to the right on each abscissa. The eccentric strengths would have to be determined with the person resisting the ergometers (which would be driven backwards by an external power supply) and the maximal forces (strengths) would be even greater than in the isometric condition.

2. Comparable fatigue curves for isometric and eccentric exercise would presumably lie appropriately higher than the curves shown, indicative of greater capacities for endurance in these exercise forms.

3. The present curves are for individual velocities (because of the predetermined contraction rate or rpm). Altering velocity would alter metabolic and related physiological demands and, thereby, the endurance potential at each power level.

4. Lastly, fatigue curves are obtained with the cooperation and enthusiasm of the person being tested. The intercepts and curves can be altered markedly by changes in the person's motivation.

IMPROVEMENT OF CAPACITIES
FOR STRENGTH, ANAEROBIC POWER, AND AEROBIC POWER

With regard to the development of any physiological capacity, it can be said that the appropriate mechanisms must be stressed by vigorous physical activity. The enhancement of strength or endurance will not be brought about by massage, dietary supplements, effortless exercise systems, or transcendental meditation.

Further, the stress must be of high intensity relative to the functional capacity to be developed. Strength exercises must be at resistances equivalent to high percentages of the maximal force. Programs to develop maximal oxygen uptake (or aerobic power capacity) must include vigorous exercise involving large muscle groups, so as to elicit change markedly different from that which accompanies daily function. As a general rule, if the level of stress of a functional capacity underestimates the initial level by much under 50%, one should not expect marked improvement.

Strength

Strength was defined as the maximum effective force for a specific body movement. Muscle bulk or, more specifically, physiological cross-sectional area, has been observed to have a direct and strong relationship to strength capacity. While no direct evidence exists for an increased number of muscle cells as a result of strength training, it is assumed that the increase in bulk is related to an increased cross-section of individual fibers. The latter would be attributable to an increase in number and/or size of the myofibrils, with actin and myosin filament density remaining constant.

Empirical evidence from physiatrists, physical therapists, and exercise program participants together with the results of controlled studies (*1, 4–6, 16–18, 20, 22, 30, 31*) leads to the following recommendations:

1. To increase the strength of a movement, exercise at very high intensity or force levels relative to the maximal (e.g., the 1 RM). One might hypothesize a minimal stimulus of 50% of the 1 RM—but it seems clear that the closer to 100% the faster the development and the greater the end result.
2. Bouts of this intensive exercise should be repeated but not necessarily for great numbers of repetitions. While the exact numbers of repetitions and the number of bouts per week for optimal development constitutes a complete unknown, something on the order of 2 or 3 bouts of 6 to 10 repetitions performed once a day (or at least every other day) is sufficient for each particular movement.
3. Strength development is a slow process. It may take months to bring about marked improvement.
4. As with most physiological capacities, the person in poorest condition relative to personal genetic limits will enjoy the most marked improvement and rate of increase (until they arrive at higher and more typical strength levels).
5. Strength should be assessed regularly (e.g., weekly) so changes in maximal resistances can be determined. If strength gains are observed, optimal development will be brought about in weight training programs by resetting exercise intensities at suitably higher levels.

The comparative effectiveness for strength training of concentric, isometric, and eccentric contractions is not known. Ergometers for eccentric contractions, however, involve considerable expense. Devices that control speed but permit maximal force expression throughout the full range of a movement (isokinetic) appear to be physiologically sound. Because of the changes in mechanical advantage that occur in a weight-lifting maneuver, the resistance for standard concentric exercise is determined by what the muscles can perform at the single point in the range at which the effective force of the movement is lowest.

It would seem that more information should be available concerning strength training, since so many persons are interested for so many different purposes—from patient rehabilitation to Olympic competition. Research in strength training is made extremely complex by a number of factors, including the recruitment and control of large groups of test subjects, the makeup of the groups obtained in terms of representing the general population, the time required for improvement, the myriad possibilities for combinations of training routines, the need for more biochemical and morphological information, and, from the standpoint of making valid testing assessments, the psychological aspects of volitional strength expression. Therefore, we are forced to operate without specific prescriptions but with three general rules of thumb: 1) high resistance, 2) brief and intense workouts, and 3) patience.

Anaerobic Capacity

Exercise that is principally dependent upon anaerobic energy-release mechanisms is characterized by repeated contractions at extremely high intensity. In the area of competitive sports, two excellent examples of strictly anaerobic activities are football (the players average 5 sec of activity each play) and the 100-meter dash. As was pointed out earlier, however, the anaerobic mechanisms are also believed to play prominent roles in physical performance in exercise that can be endured for from 2 min to at least 10 min, and to play a decreasing but still significant role in even longer bouts.

The mechanisms for anaerobic energy release lie in the biochemical changes occurring inside the active muscle cells. Because research techniques for determining these microchemical changes are still crude, we must rely on empirical evidence, gained mostly from athletics, in order to base our training regimens.

Anaerobic power capacity is enhanced by repeated bouts of high stress exercise exemplified by interval training (involving short intervals). Bursts of all-out activity for 10 to 20 sec with rest intervals of equal duration are repeated for anywhere from 3 to 10 min. Following recovery period of longer duration (e.g., 5 min), the process can be repeated.

The full story of the effects of such a regimen on high-energy phosphate concentration, glycolytic enzyme activity, cell tolerance of lactate and hydrogen ion buildup, etc., is not ready to be unfolded. Questions related to the efficacy of shorter or longer bouts of exercise, repetitions per day, and weekly schedule are open for considerable conjecture.

Aerobic Capacity

The physiological factors underlying aerobic power capacity (or maximal oxygen uptake) have been elucidated to a greater extent than in the other areas discussed. An examination of selected studies can give a clear understanding of the factors related to this capacity and the specific effects of training.

To begin with, we can examine the results of the opposite extremes of conditioning exercise—cessation of training and incapacitation. In one study, in which measurements were made over a period of some years (13), elite Swedish girl athletes (swimmers) were seen to decline in aerobic capacity when their competitive careers ended. As can be seen in Figure 6, their average $\dot{V}O_2$ max was at the upper limits for their age group during the prime years of the swimmers' competitive activity (1961). Seven years later, their average lay well below the general average for Swedish women in their early twenties. In another study (34), five healthy subjects (young

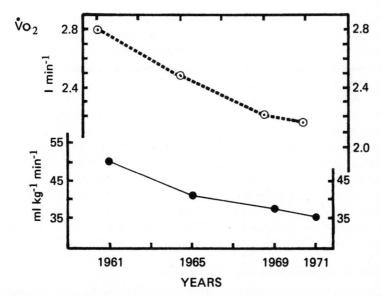

Figure 6. Average values for maximal oxygen uptake (expressed as ml per kg body weight) for elite girl swimmers tested at period of competition (1961) and years after training had been suspended (1968–69). (Figure constructed from data provided by B.O. Eriksson, Göteborg, Sweden.)

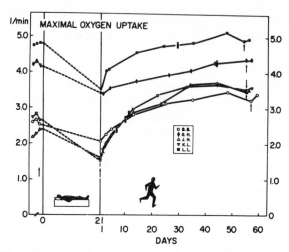

Figure 7. Values for maximal oxygen uptake for five healthy subjects before 3 weeks of bedrest, after bedrest, and during intensive training. Horizontal bars along oxygen uptake curves during training period indicate point when oxygen uptake has returned to pre-bedrest values for each individual. (Figure from Saltin et al. (*34*).)

adults) underwent a 3-week period of bedrest (i.e., an almost total lack of physical effort and no weight-bearing activity whatsoever). This was followed by an extended period of vigorous training that eventually amounted to 2 hr each day of a heavy exercise program (distance running, interval running, cycling).

In Figure 7 are presented the values for maximal oxygen uptake ($\dot{V}O_2$ max) as determined before the bedrest period, immediately after the bedrest, and at various times during the training period. All subjects dropped in $\dot{V}O_2$ max during the bedrest; the average decrease was 31% of the initial values and the greatest decrease was 46%. When training was begun, the 3 subjects who were initially in the poorest condition (lowest $\dot{V}O_2$ max) regained their pre-bedrest levels in a short period of time (see vertical bars in figure) and went on to even greater levels. For two subjects, the increases from post-bedrest to final values exceeded 100% (a doubling of $\dot{V}O_2$ max).

Physiological Changes and Aerobic Capacity

An examination of the results of these studies together with various others (*8–11, 15, 19, 25–28, 32, 33, 35, 38*) demonstrates certain patterns. For one thing, it is evident that age has an important bearing on the physiological effects of $\dot{V}O_2$ max conditioning.

Aerobic training of two months duration and longer in prepubescent children elicits increases in maximal stroke volume and maximal minute volume of cardiac output as well as oxygen extraction (arterio-venous oxygen difference across the active muscle tissue). Blood volume is increased and, as hemoglobin concentration is not altered, total circulating hemoglobin is also increased. There are further indications that heart volume, blood volume, and lung volumes (e.g., vital capacity and total lung capacity) can increase and, in this age group, remain increased throughout life. All increases described are, of course, over and above the expected natural increases with normal growth. (9, 12)

In young adults, the initiation of aerobic training results in increased maximal stroke volume, minute volume, and, to a lesser extent, oxygen extraction. Blood volume is increased with a concomitant increase in total hemoglobin (as with prepubescents the hematocrit is unchanged). Heart volume is increased with time, although this change is apparently a transient condition dependent upon maintained stress (i.e., continuation of the conditioning program).

Aerobic conditioning for middle-aged adults brings about increases in maximal stroke volume and minute volume. Oxygen extraction shows little or no change. Heart volume does not increase if such conditioning was not experienced earlier in life. Blood volume and total hemoglobin are increased with long-term training but to a lesser degree than with the younger age groups.

In both young adults and middle-aged adults, lung volumes appear unchanged even by long-term training. This includes vital capacity, total lung capacity, timed vital capacity, and pulmonary membrane diffusing capacity.

Aerobic Training and Extrafusal Muscle Fibers

Virtually all of the physiological results of conditioning programs reported in the preceding paragraphs were related to the circulatory system and, therefore, oxygen transport. As was mentioned previously, controversy exists as to whether the oxidative capacities for energy release of the extrafusal fibers themselves can be limiting under certain or all circumstances.

The most important observation that raises the argument is that, in muscle biopsies of humans, conditioning programs have brought about increases in the oxidative enzymes of the muscle cells (14). Whether or not an increased capacity of the Krebs cycle was essential to increased aerobic performance of the individual or merely an accompanying development remains an unanswered question.

Conditioning Programs for Aerobic Power Capacity

In order to increase maximal oxygen uptake, the oxygen transport system should be challenged with exercise demanding a minimum of 50% of a person's $\dot{V}O_2$ max. As with other physiological capacities, the efficacy of a low level of stress, such as 50% of maximal, will depend on the person's initial level of condition. It should prove somewhat effective for a person in poor condition but ineffective for persons in higher states of fitness.

Further, the higher the intensity is set in relation to the 50% level, the faster will be the improvement in $\dot{V}O_2$ max and the greater the eventual change. In the case of aerobic capacity, exercise intensities can be chosen that not only approach and attain $\dot{V}O_2$ max (100%) but that actually exceed it (i.e., a combination of aerobic and anaerobic energy release).

The number of exercise bouts per session, the influence of recovery periods, the mixture of intensities employed, the daily program, the number of sessions per week, etc., again present a mixed bag. From the studies performed, the following guidelines can be presented for conditioning in the general population:

1. Exercise involving large groups of muscles (e.g., running, swimming, cycling, rowing, cross-country skiing) should be employed in the range of 50 to 100% of $\dot{V}O_2$ max. The highest intensities can be employed by the highly motivated, those with no cardiac risk factors, and those with high goals!
2. No fewer than 2 sessions per week. Every other day is a preferable objective.
3. A time investment of 45 min of activity per session seems to be both highly effective and, also, practical from the standpoint of the time demands of daily life. The minimum requirement probably lies near 15 min of activity per session.

Comparing the results of a variety of conditioning studies in graphic format, we can look at the above recommendations in terms of expected results. Persons of all age groups exercising 3 times per week for 45 min each session could expect after 2 months training the results portrayed in Figure 8. As explained in the figure legend, average expected improvement is plotted against initial level of fitness with the program intensity as a major consideration. The basic observations are as follows:

1. Persons of low initial fitness could expect an average increase of 10% by employing a program of moderate exercise, 25% with high intensity exercise, and 40% with "superhigh" intensity exercise.

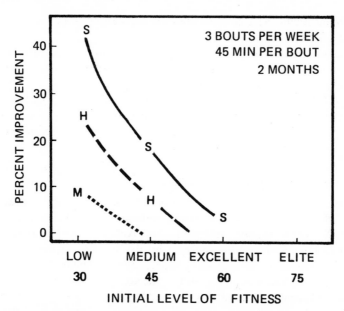

Figure 8. Improvement of aerobic capacity (expressed as percent of initial values) for three programs of exercise of various intensities for groups of varying degrees of initial fitness (designated as low, medium, excellent, and elite). All programs involve 3 sessions per week with 45 min of activity per session. Training intensities are designated as moderate, high, and superhigh and correspond to activity eliciting 50–70%, 70–90%, and 90–100% of maximal oxygen uptake, respectively. Values for initial level of fitness (30-45-60-75) are determined as maximal oxygen uptake in ml/min per kg body weight.

2. Persons of medium level fitness could expect a 10% increase with a high intensity program and a 20% increase with superhigh intensity. A moderate intensity program would be insufficient to maintain their level of fitness.

3. Persons in excellent physical condition would have to employ a superhigh intensity program in order to maintain their level of fitness. Lower intensity programs would result in a loss of aerobic condition.

4. For persons in the elite category (e.g., Olympic distance runners), 45 min 3 days a week of any intensity would constitute an inadequate program of training.

It should be remembered that the curves represent averages and, for any population, there would be a wide variation above and below the lines for individuals included. Further, the figure was constructed to include a wide age range. The younger the age group the greater the potential for development and the higher the constructed lines should be set. For older persons, the lines should be set lower.

Lastly, the abscissa was set to cover a wide range of aerobic fitness and not with any sort of even distribution of population in mind. The vast majority of persons in the general population would fall in the range of "low fitness." The next largest grouping would fall in the range of "medium fitness." A relatively small number would be classified as in an "excellent" state of fitness and the elite group would number one person for some hundreds of thousands population.

Exercise Intensities Dependent on Substrate Supply

At any level of fitness (in terms of a person's aerobic capacity), there is a range of exercise intensities in which endurance is limited by the availability of energy-yielding substrate for the oxidative mechanisms. Glucose and free fatty acids can be delivered by the blood and taken up by the muscle cells in order to successfully support exercise intensities of approximately 60% of $\dot{V}O_2$ max and lower (for the average person).

At intensities of 65% of $\dot{V}O_2$ max and higher, the limitations of uptake from the blood of needed substrate require the active extrafusal fiber to turn in increasing degree to substrate already stored (endogenous). Because the fiber has little fat storage, it turns to stored carbohydrate (endogenous glycogen). The higher the intensity, the higher the rate of endogenous glycogen utilization and depletion. Figure 9 presents the relationship of rate of glycogen depletion to relative exercise intensity (% of $\dot{V}O_2$ max) for subjects in medium to excellent levels of fitness.

Exercise intensities of 65 to 85% of $\dot{V}O_2$ max (and slightly higher for endurance athletes) can be maintained for long periods of time (e.g., 60 to 240 min) and exhaustion occurs simultaneously with glycogen depletion (concentration at or near zero) in the exercising muscles (*21, 36*). Endurance at higher intensities of exercise is limited by other factors but, in this range, endurance appears limited by endogenous substrate (therefore, glycogen).

The enhancement of initial glycogen concentration should, therefore, be of great benefit to endurance capacity in this range of high-intensity exercise. This has been born out by research (*24, 36*), which has shown that the endurance capacity of individuals exercising at similar relative intensities (in the range of 65 to 80% of their personal aerobic capacities) is directly related to the initial level of glycogen. It has been well demonstrated (*3, 24, 36*) that the glycogen storage can be markedly affected by combinations of diet and training regimen.

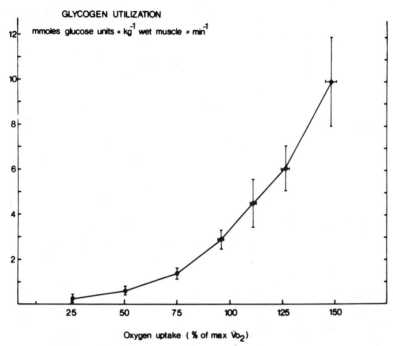

Figure 9. Relationship of rate of glycogen utilization in leg exercise to intensity of exercise (relative to percent of maximal oxygen uptake). (Figure from Saltin and Karlsson (*37*).)

SPECIFICITY OF TRAINING

As a concluding comment, the following statements can be presented for re-emphasis:

1. Physical fitness is *not* a general quality; specific capacities set limits on specific types of physical activity.
2. In order to improve a particular physical performance, the specific capacities must be identified and stressed with appropriate exercise.
3. The greater the level of appropriate stress, the greater the improvement of the level of fitness for a particular physical performance.

LITERATURE CITED

1. Asmussen, E. 1949. Training of muscular strength by static and dynamic muscle activity. 2:a Lingiaden 1949 Kongressen. Lund: Berlingska boktryckeriet.

2. Asmussen, E., O. Hansen, and O. Lammert. 1965. The relation between isometric and dynamic muscle strength in man. Comm. Dan. Nat. Ass. Inf. Paral. No. 20. 11 p.
3. Bergström, J., L. Hermansen, E. Hultman, and B. Saltin. 1967. Diet, muscle glycogen, and physical performance. Acta Physiol. Scand. 71:140–150.
4. Bonde-Petersen, F. 1960. Muscle training by static, concentric, and eccentric contractions. Acta Physiol. Scand. 48:406–416.
5. Bonde-Petersen, F., J. Graudal, J.W. Hansen, and N. Hvid. 1961. The effect of varying the number of muscle contractions on dynamic muscle training. Int. Z. Angew. Physiol. 18:468–473.
6. DeLorme, T.L. 1945. Restoration of muscle power by heavy resistance exercise. J. Bone Joint Surg. 27:645–667.
7. Edström, L., and B. Ekblom. 1972. Differences in sizes of red and white muscle fibers in vastus lateralis of musculus quadriceps femoris of normal individuals and athletes. Relation to physical performance. Scand. J. Clin. Lab. Invest. 30:175–181.
8. Ekblom, B. 1969. Effect of physical training on oxygen transport system in man. Acta Physiol. Scand. (Suppl.) 328. 45 p.
9. Ekblom, B. 1969. Effect of physical training in adolescent boys. J. Appl. Physiol. 27:350–355.
10. Ekblom, B. 1970. Effect of physical training on circulation during prolonged severe exercise. Acta Physiol. Scand. 78:145–158.
11. Ekblom, B., P.-O. Åstrand, B. Saltin, J. Stenberg, and B. Wallström. 1968. Effect of training on circulatory response to exercise. J. Appl. Physiol. 27:518–528.
12. Eriksson, B.O. 1972. Physical training, oxygen supply, and muscle metabolism in 11–13 year old boys. Acta Physiol. Scand. (Suppl.) 384. 48 p.
13. Eriksson, B.O., I. Engstrom, P. Karlberg, B. Saltin, and C. Thoren. 1971. A physiological analysis of former girl swimmers. Acta Paed. Scand. (Suppl.) 217:68–72.
14. Gollnick, P.D., R.B. Armstrong, B. Saltin, C.W. Saubert, W.L. Sembrowich, and R.E. Shepherd. 1973. Effect of training on enzyme activity and fiber composition of human skeletal muscle. J. Appl. Physiol. 34:107–111.
15. Grimby, G., and B. Saltin. 1971. Physiological effects of physical training. Scand. J. Rehab. Med. 3:6–14.
16. Hansen, J.W. 1961. The training effect of repeated isometric muscle contractions. Int. Z. Angew. Physiol. 18:474–477.
17. Hansen, J.W. 1963. The training effect of dynamic maximal resistence exercises. Int. Z. Angew. Physiol. 19:420–424.
18. Hansen, J.W. 1963. The effect of sustained isometric muscle contraction on various muscle functions. Int. Z. Angew Physiol. 19: 430–434.
19. Hartley, L.H., G. Grimby, Å. Kilbom, N. Nilsson, I. Åstrand, J. Ekblom, and B. Saltin. 1969. Physical training in sedentary middle-aged and older men, III. Cardiac output and gas exchange at

submaximal and maximal exercise. Scand. J. Clin. Lab. Invest. 24:335–344.

20. Hellebrandt, F.A., and S.J. Houtz. 1956. Mechanisms of muscle training in man: experimental demonstration of the overload principal. Phys. Ther. Rev. 36:371–383.
21. Hermansen, L., E. Hultman, and B. Saltin. 1967. Muscle glycogen during prolonged severe exercise. Acta Physiol. Scand. 71:129–139.
22. Hislop, H.J. 1963. Quantitative changes in human muscular strength during isometric exercise. J. Am. Phys. Ther. Ass. 43:21–38.
23. Karlsson, J., F. Bonde-Petersen, J. Henriksson, and H. Knuttgen. 1975. Effects of previous exercise with arms and legs on metabolism and performance in exhaustive exercise. J. Appl. Physiol. 38:763–767.
24. Karlsson, J., and B. Saltin. 1971. Diet, muscle glycogen, and endurance performance. J. Appl. Physiol. 31:203–206.
25. Karlsson, J., P.-O. Åstrand, and B. Ekblom. 1967. Training of the oxygen transport system in man. J. Appl. Physiol. 22:1061–1065.
26. Kilbom, Å. 1971. Physical training with submaximal intensities in women: Reaction to exercise and orthostasis. Scand. J. Clin. Lab. Invest. 28:141–161.
27. Kilbom, Å., and I. Åstrand. 1971. Physical training with submaximal intensities in women: Effect on cardiac output. Scand. J. Clin. Lab. Invest. 28:163–175.
28. Knuttgen, H.G., L.-O. Nordesjö, B. Ollander, and B. Saltin. 1973. Physical conditioning through interval training with young male adults. Med. Sci. Sports 5: 220–226.
29. Komi, P.V. 1973. Measurement of the force-velocity relationship in human muscle under concentric and eccentric conditions. In S. Cerquiglini et al. (eds.), Medicine and Sport, Vol. 8. Biomechanics III. S. Karger, Basel. pp. 224–229.
30. Komi, P.V., and E.R. Buskirk. 1972. Effect of eccentric and concentric muscle conditioning on tension and electrical activity of human muscle. Ergonomics 15:417–434.
31. Müller, E.A., and W. Rohmert. 1963. Die Geschwindigkeit der Muskelkraft-Zunahme bei isometrischem Training. Int. Z. Angew, Physiol. 19:403–419.
32. Saltin, B. 1969. Physiologic effects of physical conditioning. Med. Sci. Sports 1:50–56.
33. Saltin, B. 1971. Guidelines for physical training. Scand. J. Rehab. Med. 3:39–47.
34. Saltin, B., G. Blomqvist, J.H. Mitchell, R.L. Johnson, Jr., K. Wildenthal, and C.B. Chapman. 1968. Response to exercise after bedrest and after training. American Heart Association (Monograph #23), New York.
35. Saltin, B., L.H. Hartley, Å. Kilbom, and I. Åstrand. 1969. Physical training in sedentary middle-aged and older men, II. Oxygen uptake, heart rate, and blood lactate concentration at submaximal and maximal exercise. Scand. J. Clin. Lab. Invest. 24:323–334.

36. Saltin, B., and L. Hermansen. 1967. Glycogen stores and prolonged severe exercise. *In* G. Blix (ed.), Nutrition and Physical Activity Almqvist and Wiksell, Uppsala. pp. 32–46.
37. Saltin, B., and J. Karlsson. 1971. Muscle glycogen utilization during work of different intensities. *In* B. Pernow and B. Saltin (eds.), Muscle Metabolism During Exercise Plenum Press, New York. pp. 289–299.
38. Siegel, W., G. Blomqvist, and J.H. Mitchell. 1970. Effects of a quantitated physical training program on middle-aged sedentary men. Circulation 41:19–29.
39. Singh, M., and Karpovich, P.V. 1966. Isotonic and isometric forces of forearm flexors and extensors. J. Appl. Physiol. 21:1435–1437.

EXERCISE TESTING AND CONDITIONING PROGRAMS FOR THE HEART PATIENT

L. Howard Hartley

Exercise can be used as a clinical aid for either the diagnosis or treatment of heart disease. The purpose of observing a person during exercise is to elicit abnormalities that are not detectable at rest. Exercise can also be used as a therapeutic tool, since endurance training results in physiological adjustments that are beneficial to cardiac patients. Both of these interventions are gaining propularity because the physiological principles on which they are based are most applicable to coronary artery disease, a major cause of death and disability. This chapter reviews the rationale of exercise testing and endurance training and describes the details of these procedures.

EXERCISE STRESS TESTING

Background

The diagnosis of coronary artery disease is made by demonstrating a deficient oxygen supply to the myocardium. If a portion of the heart is completely deprived of oxygen, the myocardium will die, a process called myocardial infarction. The heart is said to be ischemic if the mycardium is partially but not totally lacking in oxygen.

Ischemia may be manifested as chest pain (angina pectoris), electrocardiographic changes, abnormal rhythm of the heart beat, or cardiac dysfunction. If the disease of the coronary arteries is severe, ischemia of the myocardium may be present at rest. Other less severe cases have abnormalities detectable only during the stress of physical exercise. During a stress test, the oxygen supply is unable to meet the demands of the myocardium.

Muscular exercise augments three of the major determinants of myodardial oxygen consumption: heart rate, blood pressure, and circulating catecholamines (2). Although catecholamines cannot be easily measured, heart rate and blood pressure are quite accessible. Hence the extent of stress at which ischemia appears is usually expressed as the heart rate, blood pressure, or the product of both.

Clearance for Testing

The exercise test is a safe procedure, but certain precautions are necessary. A patient should be referred by a physician if disease is suspected. The referral should include a record of abnormalities, a list of medications, chest x-ray reports, and a copy of the electrocardiogram. Several conditions known to carry an increased risk during exercise are listed on Table 1. The final decision for allowing a patient to exercise is based upon the belief that the benefits of the procedure outweigh the risks.

Certain medications affect the results of the test. Digitalis causes changes in the pattern of the electrocardiogram and may lead to false conclusions. Propranolol causes a reduction in the heart rate response to exercise. The knowledge that the patient is taking medication is important in both the conduct and the interpretation of the exercise test.

Precautions

Careful observation of the test subject during the exercise session and provision of adequate medical coverage should be a requirement for exercise testing. Even with the utmost care, complications can and do occur. The most serious complications are cardiac standstill or myocardial

Table 1. Contraindications to exercise testing

1. Myocardial infarction more recently than 6 weeks or before recovery is complete.
2. Congestive heart failure
3. Unstable angina
   a. Changing pattern of pain
   b. Changing electrocardiographic pattern
4. Hypertension (diastolic pressure over 100 mmHg)
5. Bone or joint disease
6. Pulmonary disease
7. Acute infections

infarction. Both of these occurrences are potentially fatal, although availability of treatment by qualified personnel can dramatically reduce the mortality. The frequency of occurrence of these problems varies with the nature of the population being tested. A young and healthy population has a negligible incidence of serious complications. Although middle-aged individuals also have a low incidence of problems, the frequency of occurrence is not negligible. Data from many centers across the country indicate that the incidence is about 4 serious problems per 10,000 tests (12).

Testing Procedure

Muscular exercise can be performed in many different ways. Most reference data are for leg exercise in the upright position. The exercise may be performed on a standard step, a braked cycle ergometer, or a treadmill. Each of these devices has advantages and all of them can be used to perform a test that will yield useable information. In the experience of the author, the cycle ergometer (15) is the most desirable instrument. The bicycle is inexpensive and mobile, and the oxygen requirements for each power setting are quite predictable. This makes the collection of expired gas for respiratory exchange determination unnecessary. An example of the testing laboratory as described is presented in Figure 1.

The conduct of the test requires a testing team of two persons. One individual watches the electrocardiographic tracing and the other sets the exercise intensity, verifies the pedal rate, and monitors elapsed time. The extent of training that each of the tasks requires is a subject of some debate. Each individual must have a full understanding of the techniques and principles that are involved. The technician may be trained for the position through allied health or physical education programs. However, both the technical personnel and medical personnel, such as nurses or physicians, must be further trained to detect abnormalities and problems that are unique to this clinical testing procedure.

The minimal requirements that are necessary to provide adequate medical coverage are not rigidly defined. A physician who is familiar with cardio-pulmonary resuscitation will meet the requirements of adequate medical supervision. Specially trained nurses have an excellent record of treating patients in the coronary care unit of the hospital and their presence could also constitute adequate coverage provided they are in communication with a physician.

Attention to certain details makes the testing session an event that is pleasant for both the test subject and the testing personnel. One important detail is to advise test subject to prepare for the test. The subject should

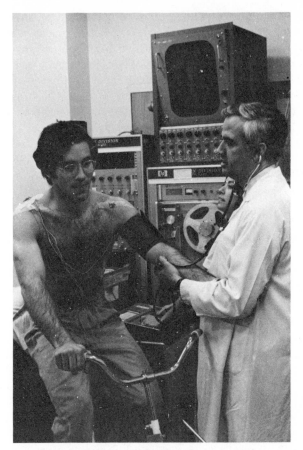

Figure 1. A laboratory for clinical exercise testing.

wear comfortable, light clothing, and comfortable shoes. No more than a light meal should be eaten within two hours of the test. The subject should be welcomed into a comfortable and clean environment with an optimal room temperature of about 21°C (70°F).

In the case of a clinical patient, an evaluation should be performed by a physician on the day of the test to be sure that the condition has not changed since the time that a referral form was filled out. This evaluation includes the history and physical examination, which should include all of the items in Table 2. A 12-lead resting electrocardiogram is taken and examined by the physician.

Table 2. History and physical
examination

History
    Chest pain
    Dyspnea
    Paroxysmal nocturnal dyspnea
    Edema
    Palpitations
    Fatiguability
    Medications
Physical examination
    Heart rate and rhythm
    Blood pressure
    Heart
    Lungs
    Extremities

After the test procedure has been explained to the subject or patient
and all questions have been answered, a consent form is signed (Sample
Form 1). Just before the exercise begins, a 6-sec strip of the electrocardiogram and the blood pressure are taken. The subject is placed on the bicycle
and the seat is adjusted to the highest comfortable position. The exercise
starts at a low power setting that is maintained for 4 min. An oscilloscope
can be used to continuously monitor the electrocardiogram. Light-weight
electrocardiographic leads are recommended because of their ease of
application and because they result in minimal motion artifact on the
electrocardiogram. The blood pressure can be taken with a standard
sphygmomanometer by auscultating over the antecubital space.

During this 4-min period, the electrocardiogram is taken every minute,
and the blood pressure is taken during the third minute. The individual
then recovers for 5 min while sitting in a chair. The test then proceeds
with 4 min of exercise at increasing power settings (usually by 25 to 50
W), which are interrupted by 5-min rest periods until the test is completed.
All heart rates, blood pressures, and symptoms that arise during the test
are recorded.

End Points of Test

There are two end points that are used by various clinicians in exercise
testing. Leg fatigue is used as an end point as, in normal persons, the time
to fatigue corresponds well to the subject's maximal oxygen uptake (10).

Table 3. End points of exercise tests

1. Chest pain
2. Dyspnea
3. Leg fatigue
4. Arrhythmias
5. Hypotension
6. Mental confusion
7. Achievement of target heart rate:
   190 − age = 85% of maximal

A second end point is a pre-selected heart rate. The author recommends an age-adjusted target heart rate equal to 85% of maximal oxygen uptake (*14*). Such a target heart rate can be determined at 190 less the subject's age in years. Various clinical indications for interrupting the test are listed in Table 3. All individuals involved in the exercise testing procedure should be aware of these signs and should stop the procedure if any one appears. Persistance of testing despite these warning signs constitutes an unneccessary risk. It is better to perform the test a second time at the particular exercise intensity if it is decided that no hazard exists rather than to ignore their appearance. The working capacity is expressed as the exercise intensity and the duration of that intensity when exercise was terminated.

Premature Beats

Premature beats occur with exercise in both normal and abnormal individuals and, hence, have little value as a diagnostic aid. They are useful in alerting the medical monitor to potential problems and exercise should be stopped if three or more premature ventricular contractions occur consecutively (Figure 2). As is implied by their name, premature beats are these which occur earlier than would be expected at the prevailing heart rate and rhythm. The electrical impulses that stimulate the heart originate in specialized tissue located in the wall of the right atrium called the sinus node. The impulse sweeps over the atrium and across a bundle of specialized tissue called the atrioventricular node and bundle of His into the ventricular wall. This impulse causes the contraction of the atria and the ventricles.

Premature beats occur before the heart is stimulated from the sinus node, and they originate from either the atria, the atrioventricular node, or the ventricular wall (ventricular premature beats or VPB's). A VPB is shown in Figure 3, and it can be identified by the following characteristics: 1) a QRS that is not proceeded by a P wave, is early, and has a different configuration than other beats, 2) an interval between the normal beats before and after the VPB that is equal to two normal beats in duration. Although these guidelines do have exceptions, they are useful in the identification of VPB's. For comparison, an atrial premature beat and an atrioventricular node premature beat are also seen in Figure 3.

Although VPB's are not diagnostic of heart disease, they may have certain features that indicate a greater likelihood of serious arrhythmias. If VPB's occur repeatedly and have more than one configuration, they are referred to as multifocal (Figure 2). If the VPB begins on the T wave of the antecedent normal beat, it is said to exhibit the R on T phenomenon (Figure 2). Two VPB's that occur together are called repetitive, and this is also shown in Figure 2. Multifocal beats, R on T phenomenon, and repetitive beats are associated with a more serious prognosis (8). Even with these three characteristics, it is not possible to diagnose heart disease on the basis of VPB's alone, but their occurrence should alert the testing monitor of impending trouble. It is important to remember that the exercise test should be discontinued if more than two repetitive beats occur together.

Interpretation of the Exercise Test

In order to interpret the exercise electrocardiogram, it is necessary to understand the principles of electrocardiography. The electrocardiograph is a galvanometer that measures the electrical potential at the surface of the body that is generated during the contraction of the myocardium. The potential is caused by the flow of charged particles into and out of the heart muscle cell (depolarization and repolarization) during the process of contraction and relaxation. The electrocardiograph is calibrated so that 1 mm of verticle deflection of the stylus is equal to 1 mV and 1 mm of horizontal distance is equal to 40 msec at the usual paper speed of 25 mm/sec.

The portions of the electrocardiogram that result from one beat are depicted in Figure 5. The P wave represents the depolarization of the atria of the heart. The QRS complex represents the depolarization of the ventricles. The ST segment is determined by the electrical potential of the myocardium after depolarization but before repolarization. The T wave is inscribed during repolarization of the ventricles. The ST segment is the portion of the tracing that is of most value in diagnosis of coronary artery disease, since it is the most likely to show changes due to ischemia.

The usual resting electrocardiogram has 12 leads. These leads were selected because they monitor the electrical activity of the heart from

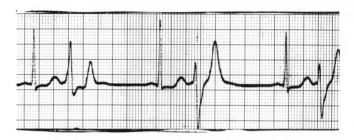

MULTIFOCAL VENTRICULAR PREMATURE BEATS

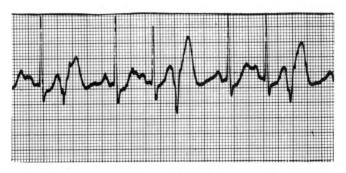

R ON T PHENOMENON

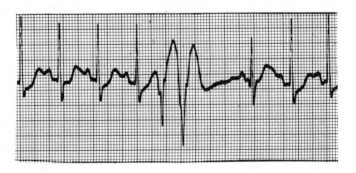

2 REPETITIVE BEATS (COUPLET)

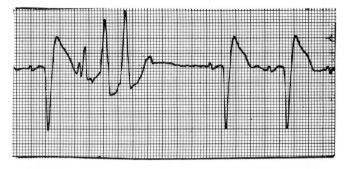

3 OR MORE REPETITIVE BEATS (VENTRICULAR TACHYCARDIA)

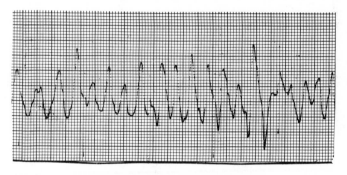

VENTRICULAR FIBRILLATION

Figure 2. Examples of ventricular arrhythmias.

different vantage points. The leads can be categorized into two types: bipolar, which measure the electrical potential between two sites on the body, and unipolar, which record the potential at one location with a reference electrode at zero potential. A full discussion of the theory behind these leads can be found in any textbook of electrocardiography.

During exercise, it is impractical to monitor and record all 12 leads and it has been reported that either lead V5 or a transthoracic lead, with one lead in the right subscapular and the other in the anterior axillary line in the fifth intercostal space, is the lead most likely to yield positive results during exercise. The recording of this one transthoracic lead is much more practical than more complex lead systems and the majority of changes that

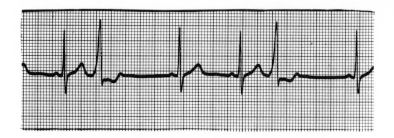

VENTRICULAR PREMATURE BEAT

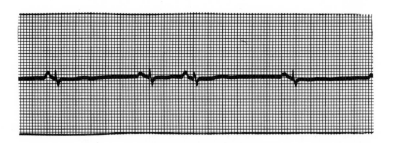

ATRIAL PREMATURE BEAT

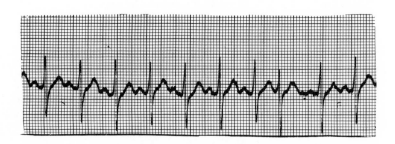

NODAL PREMATURE BEAT

Figure 3. Examples of various types of premature beats.

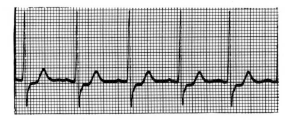

1 MILLIMETER OF ST DEPRESSION.

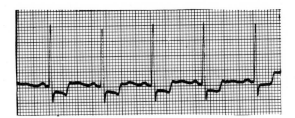

2 MILLIMETERS OF ST DEPRESSION

Figure 4. Electrocardiogram of one normal cardiac cycle.

occur with exercise can be detected (*1*). Using this lead, ST segment depression of 1 mm with a horizontal baseline (Figure 4) is strongly suggestive of coronary artery disease and more than 2 mm (Figure 4) is virtually diagnostic of myocardial ischemia (*9*).

The record of the test should include the results of the data collected at rest, during each exercise period, and for each recovery period. The reason for terminating the test should be noted. The blood pressure, heart rate, and symptoms during the test are recorded and are included in the test report. The electrocardiogram is mounted and included with the test report.

Post-Exercise Care

Following the exercise test, the patient should be observed and electrocardiogram monitored for 15 min. The final tracing should be the same as the original one, and the blood pressure should be within normal limits.

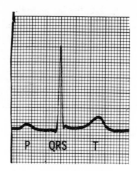

NORMAL ECG (50 MILLIMETERS/SECOND)

Figure 5. Examples of ST segment depression.

The monitor should be alert for arrhythmias occurring during the first 5 min of recovery. After the electrodes are removed, the subject may take a warm (but not hot) shower.

EXERCISE CONDITIONING FOR CARDIAC PATIENTS

The activities used for conditioning of cardiac patients usually consist of walking and jogging. Swimming has been used, but it does not allow direct access to the patient. The characteristics of the conditioning activity should include an intensity that elicits approximately 60% of maximal O_2 uptake ($\dot{V}O_2$), a duration of 30 min per session and a frequency of 3 times per week.

Such a conditioning program should result in physiological changes that are desirable for patients with coronary heart disease. The reductions in heart rate, systolic blood pressure, and blood catecholamines (6) during submaximal exercise result in a lessening of myocardial oxygen requirement. Hence, after conditioning, the electrocardiographic ST changes are less during submaximal exercise and the exercise intensity that can be achieved before angina appears is greater (7). Since improved oxygen delivery through increased collateral formation in the heart has been shown to occur only in experimental animals (4), the beneficial effects of conditioning in man are attributed to the lower myocardial oxygen requirements.

A recent report has indicated that of two groups of individuals studied, a lower incidence of coronary artery disease and a lesser mortality was found in those engaged in greater leisure time activity (*11*). There is no information to indicate whether or not the same is true in patients with coronary artery disease and it is not known if this is an effect of exercise. Elevated blood levels of cholesterol and triglycerides are known to be associated with increased incidence of coronary artery disease. As exercise conditioning has been found to lower the concentration of these lipids in the blood (*5*), exercise may contribute to a diminished risk for development of disease. Unfortunately, this effect on blood lipids is not consistently observed.

One of the most consistent observations in post-coronary programs is the improved feeling of self-confidence and well-being that the conditioning engenders. Objective measurements of psychological changes have been demonstrated (*13*). It is not surprising that psychological benefits would occur, because the patients receive such careful screening and so much attention during the conduct of the program.

A post-coronary program consists of two basic components: screening and class coverage. The screening includes exercise testing and activity prescription. The exercise testing has already been described and the results of those tests are used to determine whether an exercise program is desirable for the patient. Contraindications to endurance training are listed in Table 4. The activity that the patient undertakes should generate a heart rate that approximates 60% to 70% of maximal oxygen uptake (age-corrected) if that level can be tolerated on the bicycle test. All classes in which this activity is performed are attended by either a nurse or a physician as described under "Exercise Stress Testing."

The exercise conditioning program may be continued until satisfactory improvement has occured or until the patient shows intolerance to the exercise by developing symptoms such as chest pain or shortness of breath. A repeat exercise test is performed after 1 to 3 months to confirm that the desired physiological changes are occurring and that the cardiac status of

Table 4. Contraindications to endurance training

---

1. Myocardial infarction (until recovery)
2. Congestive heart failure
3. Unstable angina
4. Severe hypertension
5. Bone or joint disease
6. Pulmonary disease
7. Acute infections
8. Failure to tolerate exercise or testing

---

the patient has not changed. If the patient develops symptoms that are suggestive of a change in the cardiac condition, he or she should be checked by a physician before re-entering the program. In case of reasonable doubt, the patient should not be allowed to exercise until the problem is resolved to everyone's satisfaction.

The length of time that safety considerations dictate that a patient must restrict exercise to a post-coronary program is not known. Most serious events occur in the first 4 months, but they are not restricted to that time period. Hence it is recommended that patients exercise only in the presence of medical coverage. The principal problem for which medical coverage is necessary is ventricular fibrillation (see Figure 2). This arrhythmia is incompatible with life unless prompt medical treatment is administered. Defibrillation by electrical shock is almost always successful. The presence of a well-trained medical person can thus convert a potentially fatal episode into a routinely treated arrhythmia (*3*).

During the training program, attention to matters such as the temperature, bath facilities, and careful patient instruction are also important. If the exercise location is extremely hot or cold, exercise classes should be suspended. Showers should not be started for at least 15 min after the session and should not be hot. Although these points seem obvious, it is best to emphasize them to the patients. Patients should also be admonished not to exercise if they are not feeling well.

LITERATURE CITED

1. Blackburn, H., and R. Katigbak. 1964. What electrocardiographic leads to take after exercise? Amer. Heart J. 67:184–185.
2. Braunwald, E. 1971. Control of myocardial oxygen consumption. Physiologic and clinical considerations. Amer. J. Cardiol. 27: 416–432.
3. Bruce, R.A., and A. Kluge. 1971. Defibrillatory treatment of exertional cardiac arrest in seven coronary patients. J.A.M.A. 216: 653–658.
4. Eckstein, R.W. 1957. Effect of exercise and coronary artery narrowing on coronary circulation. Circ. Res. 5:230–235.
5. Gustafson, A. 1971. Effect of training on blood lipids. *In* O.A. Larsen and R.O. Malmborg (eds.), Coronary heart disease and physical fitness. University Park Press, Baltimore, London, Tokyo. p. 125.
6. Hartley, L.H., L.G. Jones, and J. Mason. 1973. The usefulness of exercise therapy in the management of coronary heart disease. *In* J.H.K. Vogel (ed.), Advances in Cardiology, Vol. 9. S. Karger, Basel. pp. 174–179.

7. Kattus, A.A., W.N. Hanafie, W.P. Longmire, R.N. McAlpin, and A.U. Revin. 1968. Diagnosis, medical and surgical management of coronary insufficiency. Ann. Intern. Med. 69:114–129.

8. Lown, B., and M. Wolf. 1971. Approaches to sudden death from coronary heart disease. Circulation 44:130–135.

9. Mason, R.E., I. Likar, R.O. Berne, and R.S. Ross. 1967. Multiple lead exercise electrocardiography. Experience in 107 normal subjects and 67 patients with angina pectoris, and comparison with coronary cinearteriography in 84 patients. Circulation 36:517–526.

10. McDonough, J.R., and R. Bruce. 1969. Maximal exercise testing in assessing cardiovascular function. J. S. C. Med. Assoc. 65:(Suppl) 26–33.

11. Morris, J.N., S.P. Chave, C. Adam, C. Sirey, and L. Epstein. 1973. Vigorous exercise in leisure time and the incidence of coronary heart disease. Lancet 1:333–339.

12. Rochmis, P., and H. Blackburn. 1971. Exercise test: a survey of procedures, safety, and litigation experience in 170,000 tests. J.A.M.A. 216:1061–1066.

13. Seigel, W., G. Blomquist, and J. Mitchell. 1970. Effects of a quantitated physical training program on middle-aged sedentary men. Circulation 41:19–29.

14. The Scandinavian Committee on ECG classification. 1967. The "Minnesota Code" for ECG classification. Adaptation of the code for ECG's recorded during and after exercise. Acta Med. Scand. Suppl. 481.

15. Von Döbelin, W. 1954. A simple bicycle ergometer. J. Appl. Physiol. 7:222–224.

Sample Form 1. Sample consent form

The test which you are asked to perform consists of riding on a specially designed bicycle. The purpose of this test is to examine the response of your heart and lungs to exercise. In this way we hope to determine (1) how much work you can do, (2) how normal your heart and lungs are, and (3) if anything can be done to improve your physical condition. In order to answer all of these questions, you may be asked to come to the exercising laboratory more than once. You may, however, stop the testing at any time. The results of these tests will be valuable to your physician in assessing your state of health.

The test consists of riding a bicycle at one or more levels of difficulty. Your electrocardiogram will be monitored throughout the exercise and recovery periods. The exercise periods will be less than 10 minutes in length and usually 3 or 4 periods will be done. If it is necessary to repeat the tests, they may be performed for longer periods of time. At the end of this test you may take a warm shower but you should not take a hot shower.

It is expected that you will complete the exercise test with no complications. Because of the very uncommon, unpredictable response of some patients to exercise, unforseen difficulties may arise which would necessitate treatment. Hence, by signing this form you also consent to treatment for any medical problem which might arise during the test including hospitalization if necessary.

Complications have been few during exercise tests and these usually clear quickly with little or no treatment. You are asked to report any unusual symptoms during the test. If you are not tolerating the work well, it usually becomes apparent and the exercise is stopped. The more serious life-threatening complications are rare, on the order of less than one in 5000 tests. Mild lightheadedness and even fainting may occur, but they are not usual and disappear quickly on lying down. Other risks of injury while climbing onto or off the bicycle are possible but are rare.

In signing this consent form you state that you have read and understood the description of the test and its complications. Any questions which occurred to you have been answered to your satisfaction. Every effort will be exerted to ensure your health and safety. You enter into the test willingly and may withdraw at any time.

CONSENT
I have read the above comments and understand the explanation, and I wish to proceed with the tests.
Signed_____
Witness_____
Date_____

RECOMMENDED READINGS

American College of Sports Medicine. 1975. Guidelines for Exercise Testing and Prescription. Lea and Febiger, Philadelphia.

Åstrand, P.-O., and K. Rodahl. 1970. Textbook of Work Physiology. New York: McGraw-Hill Book Co., New York.

Carlson, F.D., and D.R. Wilkie. 1974. Muscle Physiology. Prentice-Hall, Inc., Englewood Cliffs, New Jersey.

Close, R. 1972. Dynamic properties of mammalian skeletal muscles. Physiol. Rev. 52:129–197.

Downey, J.A., and R.C. Darling. 1971. Physiological Basis of Rehabilitation Medicine. W.B. Saunders Company, Philadelphia.

Keul, J. 1973. The relationship between circulation and metabolism during exercise. Med. Sci. Sports, 5:209–219.

Lehninger, A.L. 1971. Bioenergetics (Second Ed.). W.A. Benjamin, Inc., Menlo Park, California.

Mommaerts, W.F.H.M. 1969. Energetics of muscular contraction. Physiol. Rev. 49:427–508.

Saltin, B. 1973. Metabolic fundamentals in exercise. Med. Sci. Sports, 5:137–146.

Symposium on the Physiological Basis for Human Work Performance. 1969. Med. Sci. Sports, 1:1–56.

Weber, A., and J.M. Murray. 1973. Molecular control mechanisms in muscle contraction. Physiol. Rev. 53:612–673.

Wilmore, J.H. (ed.). 1973. Exercise and Sports Sciences Reviews, Vol. 1., Academic Press, New York.

Wilmore, J.H., and J.F. Keogh (eds.). 1975. Exercise and Sports Sciences Reviews, Vol. 3. Academic Press, New York.

Index